The Wilde Way
Unleash Your Vitality

"A Doctor's Holistic Prescription for Optimal Health and Living Your Best Life"

Dr. Heather Wilde, NMD

ISBN: 979-8-9882746-8-1

DEDICATION

I dedicate this book to you. May you dedicate the reading of this book to your past and future selves.

To the self you were, who created where you are now—to the mistakes, trauma and trials that inspired you to search for more, and find solutions to your pain.

And to the person you choose to Be. Here, now, at this moment, and every day forward, because that person will determine your life's trajectory and journey.

May you sing and dance, laugh and love along the way, no matter the chaos around you. For growth is never comfortable, and it is necessary to heal deep unconscious aspects of yourself to live the life you dream of. May you commit to your Hero or Heroine's journey and recognize that your scars are beautiful. They are proof of your power to heal.

ACKNOWLEDGMENTS

To my tribe: my friends, colleagues, and loved ones. To those who journey the outer and inner worlds with me: we may be years and miles or inches and whispers apart, but we are together—in one dimension or another.

When I do my gratitude practice, there is nothing more appreciated in my life than our connection and the knowing that I have such depth, love, and richness in my community. Thank you.

To my family for giving me roots, wings, and very special brain chemistry. Thank you for inspiring me to be who I am and loving and supporting me to the best of your capabilities.

I lovingly acknowledge the once-and-future me. I acknowledge my growth and evolution and deeply appreciate my stubborn, hopeful spirit that didn't let me give up. Again and again.

Here's to the best version of me, the one who believes in magic and is brave enough to continue to choose to accept life's challenges and evolve to be my best self on a path of consciousness, connection, and self-actualization as the entire planet experiences the growing pains of the next steps in human evolution.

ABOUT THE AUTHOR

Dr. Heather Wilde is a Naturopathic Physician, educator, mother, author, speaker, naturalist, world traveler, opportunistic yogi, boundary pusher, cultural commentator, explorer of consciousness and 5D seer. Her colleagues call her a 'naturopathic renegade' and 'eclectic physician.' One of her frenemies gave her the best compliment she ever received: that she is "80% Magic and 20% woman." Dr. Wilde circumnavigated the planet with a backpack, hiked the Grand Canyon nine times, sailed down the Nile, and meditated inside the Great Pyramid—twice. She was the first woman in history to travel to Antarctica with no supplies and attended the first silent disco on the white continent. She loves adventure, great conversations, transformative relationships, traveling, reading, puzzles, children, animals, and nature. Her philosophy is that the further you get from nature, the sicker you become. She cultivates safe space and luxurious retreats to guide you in your Hero/Heroine's Journey and create a life you love living with health and Wilde Vitality.

She specializes in detoxification and environmental medicine, stress management, and optimizing a person's health so they can create their dreams with power and vision.

An expert in preventive medicine and health fundamentals, she has also mastered the high-skill procedures associated with the highest levels of integrative medicine. She has 20 years of experience with integrative oncology, chelation, environmental medicine, orthopedic and aesthetic PRP and stem Cell therapies, sports performance optimization, bio-identical Hormone replacement, diabetes, heart disease, autoimmune diseases, and chronic disease management. Experience has shown that a solid health foundation is critical. You can do IVs, PRP, chelation, and hormone replacement, but none will optimally work if you don't have a strong nutritional and lifestyle foundation.

Her practice now concentrates on empowerment through education so people can remember who they are and what they want and have the power and vitality to create a life they love to live. One must not only support optimal body function through lifestyle elements like sleep, stress management, exercise, diet, advanced supplementation, and detoxification but also take control over mental factors, limiting beliefs, and unconscious patterns formed in childhood that form barriers to our optimal life and wellness.

She created an extensive foundational program that combines lifestyle elements and detoxification to educate and empower people to live their best lives. Take control of your health adventure at www.NaturopathicMD.com.

THE FOREWORD

Life.

You only get one.

All of us humans find ourselves at crossroads, crises, epiphanies, dead ends, and all manner of changepoints throughout life. If you are like me, you may have had more than you can actually remember...

Every day we have the opportunity to choose what to do with our time on earth, with our happiness, effectiveness, joy, fulfillment, desires, vocation, and plans. The meeting of our crossroads and decisions about our lives can be times of extreme growth and positive change or times when we freeze, stall out, regress, or even quit.

My suspicion is that if you are reading this book, you are interested in the 'way through' to a better you—a way to a better, more joyful, and more fulfilling life. Congratulations! As a veteran of many wonderful and also terrible life experiences and changes (a benefit of a long life), I know firsthand how much the decisions mean at these crossroads. I've made every kind of decision you could imagine...

Why this book? Why Dr. Wilde?

I've known Dr. Wilde for over twenty years since she was a medical student, and I was one of her professors. I've seen her pass through many change points. In fact, when she says, "Four years ago, I burned down my life," she is not engaging in hyperbole. I've seen her mature as a physician, friend, mother, family member, and probably a few other things. I've also known many people who "burned their lives down" and did not emerge in a better place.

Dr. Wilde is an example of someone who sought a deeper meaning in the pain and chaos that bring crossroads in life and found the hard-won gems that create meaningful change. Really.

This book is laid out to teach you where to look and what to consider as you move through your own crossroads. Deeper looks into why you need change, where to find it, how it often hides from us, and what to actually do are laid out here. It's real, sometimes raw, always loving, and without bullshit.

As someone who probably has made the most mistakes at crossroads, one can take it from me and use this roadmap to make the process as "you-friendly" as it can be.

Peace.

Dr. Paul S. Anderson

Physician, Author, Professor, and crossroads veteran

Contents

Dedication i

Acknowledgments ii

About The Author iii

The Foreword..v

Part I: It Is All About You 1

Introduction 2

Chapter 1: Become Embodied And Discover Yourself 4

Chapter 2: You Deserve To Thrive 10

Chapter 3: Find The Cause 13

Chapter 4: Who Are You? The Good, The Bad, And The Unconscious..16

Chapter 5: Master Your Motivation - Remember Your Why! 27

Part II: It's Complicated 38

Chapter 6: Pharmocracy 39

Chapter 7: The Power Of Lifestyle 52

Chapter 8: Stress..56

Chapter 9: Inflammation 62

Chapter 10: Toxicity 69

Part III: The Wilde Way To Detox 95

Chapter 11: How To Detox 96

Chapter 12: How To Choose The Best Way To Detox..............106

Part IV: How To Live Your Best Life......................................112

Chapter 13: You Are What You Eat: Don't Be Fake, Fast, Cheap, Easy, Or Toxic..113

Chapter 14: MYA 126

Chapter 15: Invest In Sleep And Thrive 136

Chapter 16: Detox Your Home By Choosing Clean Products ...146

Chapter 17: Mindset - Emotional Detox................................157

Chapter 18: Digital Detox...169

Chapter 19: Daily Detox Boosts 183

Chapter 20: Don't Forget Vitamin N 202

PART I
IT IS ALL ABOUT YOU

INTRODUCTION

Four years ago, I blew up my life.

After crying and lying around in my own misery for a few years, I committed to the process outlined in this book, continued to do the work, and I am living my best life, most of the time. You can, too, if you implement the processes and knowledge shared in this book.

You were born into the most magnificent machine in the known Universe, but no one taught you how to take care of it properly. For that reason, consider this book as a user's manual for Optimal Quantum Powered Mystical Meat Suit Wellness. Reading this book will be one of the best health decisions you have ever made because it is an innovative guide to health and vitality and a compilation of the best resources available to survive and thrive in the 21st Century.

You have begun an incredible "Choose Your Health Adventure" and have the opportunity to make the most important commitment of your life – the commitment to be healthier, happier, and more invested in your wellness. Implementing what you learn in this book will treat the three main causes of chronic disease and accelerated aging: stress, inflammation, and toxicity. This book was designed to accompany The Wilde Vitality Detoxification Program, the most advanced detoxification and wellness course you can do in the comfort of your own home and without a prescription. The knowledge shared in this book is powerful and effective when you apply what you learn to your daily life, even without the full course. Here's a little bit about me. My name is Dr. Heather Wilde, and I am a Naturopathic

Medical Doctor who has been practicing environmental and functional medicine for 20 years. This book is a compilation of what I have learned in the laboratory of my own body, while researching difficult patient cases, writing articles, consulting with patients, and studying with some of the most brilliant minds at the forefront of 21st-century medicine.

If you want more energy, better sleep, a more positive outlook on life, an improved mood, mental clarity, balanced hormones, less pain, regulated digestion, an optimally functioning hormonal and immune system, and a healthier, stronger, more beautiful body, read on. If you commit to this process and take action, trust me, it will revolutionize your life.

CHAPTER 1
BECOME EMBODIED AND DISCOVER YOURSELF

What does it mean to "Live your best life?"

Do you even know?

For most of my life, I didn't.

I was running from one lover to another, jumping jobs, letting the bridges I burned light my way, drinking and playing cards every night of the week, suppressing my emotions with addictions, barely paying attention to when I was hungry, thirsty, in pain, upset, or tired.

Eventually, I developed a crazy heart arrhythmia, much of my hair fell out, I started having hot flashes and uncontrollable panic attacks. It was a wake-up call I could no longer ignore, and I decided it was time to stop believing I was invincible.

I looked at my life and saw that if I wanted to have a healthy, happy, and fulfilling second half of my life, it was important for me to actually do some self-analysis, self-care, and self-love, or my body would become a prison. I have done the work; I have walked the walk, and I can share my wisdom gathered from almost killing myself with work, unhappiness, stress, and bad habits.

If I could choose one concept for you to fully integrate and apply from this book, it would be for you to be present with your body, pay attention to YOU, and how you honestly feel when you do certain behaviors. When you increase awareness around how you have created your current results, you can commit to creating something different. When you consciously respond to hardships differently, more positively, you reprogram yourself with an upgraded default operating system designed to ensure your success.

Be unabashedly embodied. Recognize what you have created for yourself, recognize that you do have the power to get different results, set your intention, and do something different.

How do you feel?

What do you like?

Who do you want to be?

What do you want?

It's okay not to have all the answers now, but I promise you, the answers will come to you.

I recently recognized that I did everything our culture told me I 'should' do to be happy. I went to an Ivy League school, got a doctorate in an innovative scientific service field that revolutionizes lives, started a business, married a tall, handsome doctor, got purebred dogs, started a family, worked a lucrative corporate job, wore designer clothes, and drove a safe car.

I was walking with my son and his father along the beach in Orange County in the summer of 2017.

I said to my son's father, "I understand why the French say '*Je suis content.*' I am happy."

I was content. Everything was nice. It was all fine—pretty OK.

Less than a year later, my life had blown up. I lost my corporate job, was sued twice, started a new business, my brother was hospitalized, my dog died, I had a huge falling out with my family, my cat died, my doctor found precancerous lesions, and I filed for divorce.

It was like the Universe said, "Content? No way, girl, you want to say, 'Laissez les bon temps rouler!' Let the good times roll, Cherie!"

The journey to the other side of that experience was not easy. There were times of extreme despair, and I sat in my backyard, got high, and compulsively read fantasy romance novels for more days than I would like to admit. I didn't eat, move, or feel hope or excitement, and I was alone and isolated most of the time. In hindsight, the experience helped me to erase many of the layers and masks I had built over my true self, and when I chose to peel them off one by one, I unveiled my more authentic self and I became someone else. I became authentically me.

I created a new life, one that evolves more and more into 'My Best Life.' I can honestly feel gratitude for the 'bad' and the 'ugly' because I proved to myself the truth of *"what doesn't kill you, really does make you stronger,"* if you choose to allow for it to do so.

I got real with myself about whether I wanted to lie down, give up, take prescriptions for anxiety, depression, and fibromyalgia, and numb out in mediocrity and artificial reality for the rest of my life. Or did I want to get up, examine my shadow, make different choices, and embrace every moment of the incredible miracle called life?

If you open yourself up to the experiences of your life, unadulterated by booze and screens, food and porn, prescriptions, Netflix, shopping, drama, and social media, you will eventually be awed by what you find in the mirror.

It is, indeed, beautiful.

I hope that you are present with yourself when you look in the mirror (literally AND metaphorically). May you have the courage to go to the dark places that scare you, to shine the light of love and forgiveness, and to let go of your old story. I hope you let go of your old life with gratitude and become brave enough to create something that makes your heart sing. I wish for you to wake up in the morning and feel something to the effect of, *"Hot DAMN, I get another day of awesomeness and adventure and juicy amazing authentic moments, and I feel so good, and I am excited to see what this day brings to me so I can learn more about who I am and how I am consciously creating my life!"*

Most of the time anyway.

I heard somewhere that life is 10% what happens to you and 90% how you choose to react to the shit-tastic fucknado you may find yourself in. Choose wisely. Choose happy. Choose healthy. Choose to live your best life.

If you are having health issues, your body is trying to communicate that something is out of balance, and if you don't pay attention to it and change your behavior, it will likely get worse. It isn't as simple as driving a different car, getting a new job, or starting a new love relationship. It is about building a relationship with yourself, committing to yourself, and taking care of your health and happiness. Your body is sending you signals. Decipher the code it is transmitting. Pick up what it is putting down.

"The body is always telling you something.
Nine times out of ten, you are ignoring it."
~Dr. Anna Kate Cascio

Remember, no one else can 'fix' or 'heal you.

Your health adventure depends on you and only you. I designed this process to empower you to take control of your health and body with deceptively simple lifestyle changes coupled with knowledge of emerging medical research. This combination will transform your entire life for the better. You will be clearer, more confident, truer to yourself and your dreams, and probably more authentic than you have been since you started learning to please others before you please yourself. When you choose 'all in,' this is a life-altering journey.

As a practicing naturopathic physician and functional medicine doctor for 20 years, I have seen diseases become more complicated and difficult to resolve. People have higher levels of toxicity, more emotional stress, and rampant inflammation. Chemical toxicants and pollutants are everywhere. It can be overwhelming and even demoralizing when you start to pay attention. You may have heard about 'toxins' and 'detoxes,' but the more appropriate term is 'toxicant' when referring to chemicals from industrial sources. Bacteria, molds, and other living organisms make toxins, and chemical companies make toxicants. Harmful toxic exposures that affect modern people aren't just restricted to chemical forms; you are inundated with toxic influences from social interactions between friends, family, frenemies, and strangers, as well as physical exposure to radiation and electromagnetic frequencies. Forget what you've heard before from very expensive marketing teams. Deep, effective detoxification is not just a simple matter of going on a juice diet, taking a magic pill, or putting your feet in a detox bath. To really shift your life in a meaningful and discernable way, you will need to re-examine the kind of life you are living and conduct a complete detoxification of your experience. By using a holistic method to detox, you will be able to live life to the fullest, break free from all that does not serve your highest and best, and enjoy vibrant health so you can move confidently in the direction of your dreams with clarity and power. It is my belief that we are all on this planet to live lives that bring our hearts joy and fulfillment. I think we all have something unique that will bloom out of our experiences and add to the tapestry of humanity as a whole. I became a doctor because I believe that people deserve to thrive. If you can assist a person to shift their experience of their life into a more positive one, you improve an entire universe of existence. You are a product of your genetics and environment, and the sad truth is that you have probably allowed cultural mores, learned patterns, and negative mindsets to grow unchecked and create a default operating system that has clouded your view of your purpose.

It is no surprise that you may be simply going through the motions. Hour to hour, day to day, and moment to moment, you move through life with no clear direction, no real engagement, trying to survive and wrestle some shallow happiness out of your existence.

Choose a different adventure.

Choose to cut through the fog.

Choose to overcome your past trauma and write a new story.

Bask in the sunlight of purpose, clarity, health, vitality, and meaning.

You only live once—in this body, anyway. So why not choose to make it your best life?

CHAPTER 2
YOU DESERVE TO THRIVE

In Western cultures, sickness has traditionally been defined as physical, medical, or, more recently, mental. Western psychology and psychiatry have progressed quite a bit over the years and are no longer regularly doing frontal lobotomies or hysterectomies on unhappy women. Now antidepressants are prescribed at an incredible rate. According to the National Institutes of Health, the number of antidepressants prescribed per year has increased by 300% in the last 20 years. People are more and more unhappy and desperate to no longer feel that way. Unfortunately, antidepressants don't really work to fix the problem; they just dull your feelings. Did you know that for an antidepressant drug to be deemed 'effective,' it only has to work 50% of the time for 50% of the patients it is prescribed to? Yikes. Many people think the withdrawal symptoms from stopping the antidepressants that don't actually work are their "depressive symptoms," and they go back on the medication that numbs them out and sets them up for long-term issues. There must be another way.

Believe me, there is. However, conventional medicine has not reached the point where it is embracing the research supporting alternative medical therapies and the mind-body connection. It takes, on average, 17 years for clinical research to impact conventional medicine. I don't know about you, but I don't want to wait for them to catch up. I built this program so YOU are educated in a holistic, practical, natural, functional, and logical way. You will know your body better and will be able to advocate for yourself and your loved ones. The word 'Doctor' is from the Latin word - *Docere* - to teach. Are you ready to learn?

We are all energy, and our thoughts and emotions impact our physical, mental, and emotional states. Why? As I answered my son, Kieran, when he was three and repetitively asked until I couldn't give another logical reason: "*Why? Why? Why Mama? Why? Why?*"

When you really get down to it, the answer is always "*Quantum Physics, Baby. Quantum. Physics.*"

Indigenous shamanic medicine, Ayurveda, and Acupuncture have effectively used holistic models of diagnosing and treating disease, sickness, and imbalances for over 5000 years. I love acupuncture because every time they have studied it with the Western mind, it proves effective. With thousands of years of experience and success, they take into account how toxicity, spiritual pollution, emotional stress, interpersonal interactions, toxic behaviors, and other factors strongly impact the human body, psyche, and overall sense of well-being.

These environmental factors may then manifest themselves in actual physical illness or impaired physical performance. You may seem perfectly 'healthy' according to conventional care and the ridiculously shallow testing they generally run. These basic lab tests will likely come out 'normal,' and your provider will likely explain it away with: "*You are just getting older*" and "*It's all in your head*" and probably prescribe an antidepressant. I disrespectfully disagree. I believe you deserve to experience vibrant health. It is a basic human right to thrive.

The United States is ranked last, compared to other affluent countries, in access to care, administrative efficiency, equality, and outcomes, despite having the most expensive medical system. It is also the only 'for-profit' medical system in the first world. The conclusion I draw from that is that you must take responsibility for and control of your own health and health care. Empower yourself through education. No one else will do it for you. It is absolutely your choice. If you don't take responsibility and make changes that impact your health in positive ways, there's a whole healthcare system waiting for you with drugs and surgery. After all, that's what it does best.

"You deserve to thrive, not just survive."
~Dr. Jesika DiCampli

Ask yourself, *"How do I feel?"* Then, *"Do I feel as well as I want to?"*

There's nothing wrong with asking this question. It is okay to want more vitality than you have. Pretending that everything is fine only ensures that your experience stays the same or worsens.

CHAPTER 3
FIND THE CAUSE

Imagine this scenario for me. You are driving in your car, and the check engine light comes on. Eventually, you will take it to a mechanic (a car doctor) to discover the problem. The check engine light is an initial "symptom." At the garage, the mechanic pokes around under the hood for a bit and then finds you to tell you not to worry; they can fix the problem with your car today. They go over to their toolbox, take out some wire snips, and cut the wire to the light. The problem is solved! The symptom is gone, the light is off, and you pay the bill.

Let me ask you: how comfortable would you be getting in that car and driving the people you love? Do you trust that the problem is solved? Would you be happy to pay that bill? Most pharmaceutical drugs merely cut the wire to the symptom light.

Unsurprisingly, many modern people can't get the relief they desire from psychopharmaceutical drugs and chemical-based medicine. When you look at the top 10 medications prescribed in the United States and Western Europe, anti-anxiety, antidepressant, anti-hypertensive, and metabolic medications like thyroid, diabetes, and cholesterol-lowering drugs are always on the list. After decades of drug and surgical interventions, cardiovascular disease still kills more Americans than any other illness.

There's something wrong here. Even though these diseases have been bombarded with a wide range of chemical cocktails over the years, Americans are still sicker and sicker, and we pay more and more money for care. There is no solution in sight other than new drugs. This is because the root causes of these diseases are not being addressed. Not biochemically, not emotionally, not spiritually, and certainly not mentally.

"Suffering is not required. There is another way."
~Dr. Lori DiBacco

People are more than their physical parts. You're not just a collection of blood pressure readings, blood sugar levels, blood counts, liver function tests, lipid panels, and biochemical indicators. These may come out unremarkable and fall within the 'normal range.' But that doesn't mean people with 'normal' labs don't feel lousy, stressed, and suffer from 'brain fog.' Do you want to get well and step away from just choosing to survive and live fully? You must look at your complete being in 'holistic' terms.

You are more than your body and genetic code. I believe the mind and spirit can heal disease. If you aren't familiar with Louise Hay and her book, *You Can Heal Your Life,* I invite you to read it. Yes, the mind and spirit are mighty and can shift the quantum energy of your body and heal you. And we still live in a 3D world beholden to nature's physical laws.

What is 'holistic' medicine? Just as your mind is composed of more than your brain, your life and overall health are composed of more than just your body. What you eat, how you construct and experience your day, and what environments you find yourself in are all part of your holistic health. My health philosophy and practice of medicine are holistic.

I perform advanced functional laboratory testing to find the root 'physical' cause of disease or dysfunction, identify and enact lifestyle changes, and provide personalized supplementation solutions while recommending meditation and addressing the other emotional and energetic factors. The human organism and experience go beyond the physical. While biochemistry and your physical body are important, they are not the complete picture. Far from it.

When medicine starts looking at people as more than just physical data, it will make progress toward effective treatments. When it ceases to be so reductionist, breaking people down into different body systems and ignoring that the immune system is affected by the digestive system connected to the nervous system, and so on, it will be closer to a 'health care' system.

Did you know that many cases of depression are due to hypothyroid? But psychiatrists don't often run thyroid labs; that's the realm of endocrinologists, and the best therapy isn't utilized because the provider has too narrow a view. There's a lack of understanding of holism in Western medicine. Whatever you are suffering from, whatever physical manifestations of stress or lack of purpose may be hounding you, whatever aches and pains you may experience, all of these can be addressed most effectively with a holistic approach.

CHAPTER 4
WHO ARE YOU? THE GOOD, THE BAD, AND THE UNCONSCIOUS

According to Carl Jung, the human mind is poetically described as an iceberg consisting of two parts: the conscious mind and the unconscious mind. We are only aware of what is above the water and what can be seen, i.e., our 'conscious' mind, the part of us aware of our thoughts, feelings, and perceptions in the present moment. It is the mind that makes decisions, solves problems, chatters endlessly to itself all day, and creates our sense of self.

The unconscious mind is the other 90% of who we are; it is below the water, and we largely have no idea what it is up to. It is the part of the mind that operates outside of our awareness and contains our unconscious thoughts, feelings, and memories. It is the source of our instincts, impulses, and automatic responses.

Jung believed that the conscious and unconscious minds interact to create human behavior. He theorized that the unconscious mind communicates with the conscious mind through dreams, symbols, and other unconscious expressions. Jung also believed that the unconscious mind is constantly striving to balance the conscious mind by expressing repressed or suppressed emotions and thoughts. This balance is crucial for psychological well-being and can be achieved through a process of 'individuation,' where the individual integrates their unconscious material into their conscious awareness.

"It is the truth that heals."
~Dr. Bill Mitchell

The creation of the unconscious mind is a complex process that begins at the moment of birth and continues throughout the lifespan. It is shaped by various factors, including genetics, environment, and experience. In child development, the first seven years of life are particularly significant in the creation of the unconscious mind. During this time, the brain is rapidly developing and forming neural connections, and children are exposed to a wide range of experiences and stimuli.

These experiences and stimuli are stored in the brain and can shape the child's unconscious mind in two ways. Firstly, they can form schemas, which are mental frameworks that organize and categorize experiences. Schemas serve as the building blocks of the unconscious mind and can influence how children process and interpret new information. They are filters through which you interpret everything you experience.

Secondly, experiences and stimuli can shape the development of unconscious beliefs, attitudes, and emotions. These unconscious processes can be thought of as a default operating system that will influence behavior and decision-making without conscious awareness throughout a person's lifespan. Neurons that fire together write together, creating superhighways of information in the brain.

Herein lies the crux of our modern human struggle. It is why some of us eat our feelings while others sabotage themselves with high-risk behaviors that are not beneficial to us. Negative emotions and experiences can trigger an unconscious pattern or strategy that then drives your behavior down that superhighway that was built when you were three and your mother gave you a cookie to stop crying.

It is no use blaming your mother, as she was doing her best with the tools she had at the time. I experienced significant healing when I recognized my parents were doing their very best and I could forgive them. Is it time to forgive yours?

You are an adult, and you have chosen to continue the behavior that is sabotaging you. You learned that behavior as a strategy for getting your needs met. It was a means of coping when you were very young, before the age of 7. You have been using those basic programs to deal with your life and meet your needs ever since. You will agree that the strategies you used when you were 6 to get your needs met do not look good on you when you are 40 years old. Are you ready to evolve and dissolve those strategies that no longer serve you?

Hypnosis, neuro-linguistic programming (NLP), psychoanalysis, shadow work, and inner child healing are all designed to bring the unconscious into the light, and that is why they are so powerful and necessary. Those tools help you become conscious of your unconscious wounds and patterns that are no longer serving you and, in doing so, release them, let them go, and be free to be the ultimate you.

Living your best life depends on living with integrity and accountability. That is where health and vitality come from. When you connect with yourself and admit responsibility for creating the life you are currently living, you can honestly face your fears and your desires. You may recognize that you are so much more than the sum of your parts. You may become aware of the gifts and resources you have and commit to the dreams you have dreamed. Remember the wishes you made upon the stars? Do you believe wishes come true and miracles happen? I do. I have seen magic with my own eyes. Miracles do not happen in a vacuum. When you compare what is manifesting in your reality to what you truly desire, you become aware of the difference. Now is a perfect opportunity to set intentions, wish on stars, pray for miracles, and create change by identifying how you can show up differently to get different results. What goals can you set? What micro-movements can you make? What can you choose to no longer do? This requires introspection, a lot of honesty, and the courage to become aware and change. There's the physical you, the biochemical you, the emotional you, the spiritual you, the psychological you, the cultural you, the relational you, and the conscious and unconscious you.

WHO ARE YOU?

When someone introduces themselves, they usually qualify themselves with a role: I am a teacher, I am a doctor, I am a mother, I am a sister, I am a daughter, etc.

"We are human beings, not human doings."
~The Dalai Lama

Unfortunately, you may depend upon those roles, those boxes you live in, to determine your place in society and your perceived worth. You may become a one-dimensional character in those roles. Are you an automaton going about your life based on an operating system you are unaware of, built by your culture and environment before you could give consent? You may not even realize you are more than the expectations, rules, and responsibilities that society and your family have programmed you with. That doesn't even come close to the beauty and complexity of what you contain inside of you.

"The mass of men (humans) lead lives of quiet desperation. What is called resignation is confirmed desperation."
~Henry David Thoreau

By resigning yourself to the expectations you were raised with, the roles you play, and the kind of identity that you have created to keep your ego safe, you forget who you are—who you wanted to be when you felt safe and secure and could dream big. This is part of why you suffer. Why are you so susceptible to stress, changing situations, and the vagaries of life? It is because you are likely not living with authenticity. You don't even know who you are anymore. You probably don't know what you want out of life. And you aren't showing up for yourselves in support of your dreams, nor are you treating yourself to the self-love and self-care you deserve.

"Alas for those that never sing, but die with all their music in them!"
~Oliver Wendell Holmes

ARE YOU GOING TO DIE WITH YOUR SONG INSIDE OF YOU?

Limiting beliefs are judgments that you make about

what you believe to be true. They limit your possibilities and success, and they most often come from your childhood upbringing. Part of your default operating system is formed from patterns you observed in your parents or caregivers and what they told you, which you then internalized and believed to be true.

Children integrate what they are told and what they experience into their unconscious minds. These limiting beliefs can hold you back in all aspects of your life and in all kinds of ways. Let me give you a personal anecdote to explain this further:

When my son was five, we went on his first camping trip to Lake Tahoe. As we were driving into the campground, the Ranger asked us if we'd ever camped in bear country before, and I replied that I had.

She pointed out that there were bear boxes to lock up our food at every campsite. I thanked her, took the map, and drove into the campground. My son was shocked. How was it possible that we were going to sleep outside when bears were around?

He had a constant litany of questions and concerns about the bears. I kept explaining to him that we didn't have anything to worry about and would be safe; we just needed to take precautions.

We set up the tent and started the fire. "*Bears, bears! Bears?*" my son said.

We roasted s'mores, and he continued to chant, "*Bears? Bears, Mama!?*"

We were in a busy campground with people all around, and he would circle back to "Bears, bears, bears!"

Hours later, we were going to sleep in the tent, and finally, I had to come up with something so he could settle down and sleep.

His favorite toy and imaginary friend for his entire life has been a little bear, BB. I went to Cornell, which has a bear as its mascot. My brothers went to Brown, which also has a bear as a mascot.

I said to him, *"Don't worry, dude. You've got bear medicine. Our family has bear medicine."*

He asked, *"What's bear medicine, Mama?"* And I replied, *"It's when the spirit of the bear recognizes itself in your spirit. And you are like family, and you don't need to fear the bear."*

He went right to sleep.

The following day, we were hiking down to the lake, and it was along a popular, paved path. We were leisurely exploring, picking up pinecones, listening to the birds, and looking at the trees. It was a beautiful summer day in California, and suddenly, about 30 yards away, walking out of the brush, I saw a bear. I have hiked all over bear country for two decades and I had never seen one in the wild before.

I used one arm to grab my son underneath his armpits and backed up while scanning both sides of the trail and using my other hand to find my knife. I was looking for cubs and planning on how best to protect my son. The bear looked at us, nodded its head like, *"Hey, bruh,"* and turned and walked away from us toward the lake.

When we had some distance between us, I took a video walking behind the bear because we were headed in the same direction.

In the video, you can hear my son saying, *"Beary!*

Beary! Look, Mama, there's the bear. Hi bear!"

I asked him later, "*Kieran, you were freaking out last night about bears, and then we saw an actual one this morning, and you weren't worried. Why not?"*

He looked at me like I was an idiot and said, "*Well, Mama, you said we have bear medicine.*"

This experience was a turning point in my parenting, not only in how I parent him but also in how I interact with and understand my own inner child. At that moment, I recognized that under the circumstances I would likely never understand, he believed something I said as an absolute truth and it became a part of his worldview and operating system.

At that moment, I committed to only speaking to him in ways that supported him in being more resilient and confident, healthy, happy, and positive. The way your parents spoke to you became your inner voice, and inspired your inner dialogue. I am more mindful of how I speak to myself and my inner child as well.

Life gives us opportunities to heal our wounds so we can thrive, and this experience helped me recognize that hurtful things said to me 30 years ago have been internalized as my truth and were unconsciously limiting what I believed I could achieve and even what I deserved. I am not new to this sort of healing journey, and every time I peel a layer back and heal, there is another waiting beneath it. I may take a break between layers, but I am committed to that healing. You may have been told you were stupid, lazy, or that you'd never amount to anything. My father told me I would never amount to anything and that I would end up eating canned tripe, homeless on the side of the road. I scoffed and replied, *"Huh, I didn't realize they can tripe."*

Even though I was older and recognized it wasn't true, I was still a child, and that poison came from a parent figure. Part of me believed it. As I continue healing, I experience old wounds surfacing. Limiting beliefs that have been part of my default operating system are coming into my awareness, ready to be reprogrammed and overcome. Becoming aware of and healing unconscious childhood programming is tremendously revolutionary and integral to "the work."

EXAMPLES OF COMMON LIMITING BELIEFS ARE:

- I'm too old.
- I'm too young.
- I don't have enough time.
- I don't have enough money.
- I'll never be successful.
- I'm not smart enough.
- I'm not good enough.
- I don't have enough willpower.
- I make a mess out of everything.

Awareness is an intrinsic ingredient of wellness. Vital, holistic health comes from looking at yourself honestly and choosing to love and forgive the pieces you previously thought were 'wrong,' 'ugly,' 'not good enough,' or 'bad.' Then, you can recognize how you got where you are and commit to making different choices. As you physically detoxify your body, emotions and automatic behaviors designed to keep you stagnant and 'safe' will come up.

I see it in every client I detoxify. Uncomfortable feelings are part of the reason you have addictions and self-sabotaging behaviors. These are the feelings you have been suppressing with those addictions to substances, distractions, and emotions like fear, helplessness, and anger.

Neurons that fire together form skills, habits, and patterns of behavior. Emotions you experience frequently can also become a pattern of behavior or an emotional addiction. I recognized recently that I was addicted to fear and anxiety, and those emotions could rise out of nowhere when I didn't expect them to give my body the emotional hit I was used to. My theory is that older adrenaline junkies suffer from anxiety because the anxiety gives them the rush they used to get from driving fast cars and jumping out of airplanes.

Emotional addiction is a form of chemicalization; an addiction to the chemicals your body produces during different emotions. You can compare it to loving the endorphins from a runner's high or adrenaline junkies searching out new risky adventures. Do you know anyone who likes being angry?

I am working on becoming unconsciously positive, rather than unconsciously stressed, anxious, and negative. My programming was built from being raised in an environment with frequent angry outbursts, fear, resentment, and relatively constant anxiety. Those emotions feel 'normal' to me and are part of my default settings. I don't enjoy that version of me. I don't, in fact, want to grow up to be my parents, and so I consciously choose healthier and happier emotions whenever I can. Being aware of what is happening psychologically and physiologically is helpful, but I haven't mastered it yet, and that is okay.

I want you to remember this story when negative emotions surface during your healing journey. They will whisper self-defeat and hopelessness to you and aim to sabotage you. They have been keeping you in the holding pattern of dysfunction, unhappiness, and the disease that you have likely been experiencing since you were a teen. They want to keep the status quo. These feelings are the triggers that activate the patterns created by your childhood experiences. They are historical programs in your default operating system, and they have served their purpose. You can now choose to let them go.

You CAN choose to heal. You CAN choose to overcome. You CAN choose to free yourself. It starts by identifying those deep, frightening feelings, shedding light on them, being mindful, reprogramming your mind and neurological patterns, and committing to showing up in love. Love and laughter, because love is always the answer, and laughter is the best medicine. You have the power to choose. You can choose for life to be a poignant, hilarious adventure; a farcical, fantastic journey. Or you can choose for it to be a negative, exhausting and frightening experience. Whatever you choose, choose to enjoy it. After all, no one gets out alive, and you may as well enjoy the ride.

"Whether you think you can or you think you can't, you're right."

~Henry Ford

CHAPTER 5
MASTER YOUR MOTIVATION -
REMEMBER YOUR WHY!

Choosing to devote time, energy, and resources to create a new default operating system for your body, mind, and emotions is something to be proud of. Take a moment and appreciate how you are showing up for yourself! Give yourself a high five, or a hug. You are doing such a good job.

Now, imagine, what does your success look like? What is the sound of success? How does it feel in your heart and body? The better you envision and integrate those sensory perceptions, the faster you reach your goals.

I want to ensure that your commitments to yourself last and have the most impact on your life. So often, people create health resolutions with the best of intentions, and they fall away within a few days or weeks. The detoxification health reset program I created teaches accountability and brain programming tricks to support you in creating a new neurology for a healthy lifestyle. As you create these new habits, I ask that you choose to commit to taking an honest look at yourself and assess what you want from life. Envision how you want to experience your best life.

Creating a new healthy life for yourself takes mindfulness about what you consume. Your consumption is more than the food and drink you put in your body. It includes what you consume with your mind through social media, screens, beliefs, relationships, etc. It is up to you to consciously eliminate things that do not serve you. What are you willing to do to feel good, and what cultural norms are you brave enough to ignore in order to thrive?

> *"Everyone has a plan until they get punched in the face."*
> **~Mike Tyson**

The physical element is at the forefront of your experience, but health starts with mental, emotional, and spiritual decisions. You may be reading this book to learn how to reverse some of the major causes of chronic disease and increase your health and longevity. Why else are you doing it? Your reasons are essential to helping propel you through this often-complex process. When the ferocious feelings that you have been suppressing for most of your life come at you in full force, remember your '*Why.*' It will give you strength and help you maintain the process.

Let's start by exploring *Why* you are doing this.

It is estimated that 45% of your daily behavior is unconscious - or automatic. That means that your unconscious mind is running behavior patterns in response to triggers - or things that elicit a behavior to happen.

You don't have to think about how to operate the car while you navigate the path to work or how to open the refrigerator to emotionally eat.

If you can identify a behavior you want to eliminate and then identify its triggers, you can recode your brain with a new habit. Let's look at what new habits you specifically wish to create in your life.

DO YOU WANT TO

- Find the optimal diet for you
- Lose weight
- Improve energy
- Improve a disease process
- Clear up skin
- Improve self-esteem
- Improve digestion
- Improve sleep
- Get rid of brain fog
- Improve the quality of your life
- Prevent or reverse disease
- Get rid of the body pain
- Improve mental outlook—relieve anxiety, depression, etc.
- Improve hormone balance
- Improve sex life
- Improve fertility

What else?

WHAT HABITS DO YOU WANT TO INSTALL TO SUPPORT YOU?

Eating healthy, whole foods and doing it mindfully

- Meditation and mindfulness practice
- Setting daily intention

- Drinking water
- Getting into the habit of exercise
- Prioritizing sleep
- Limiting exposure to media
- Taking daily supplements
- Avoiding chemical toxicants
- Positive self-talk and a happy mindset

What else?

MOTIVATION STRATEGIES

In Neurolinguistic Programming (NLP), a 'strategy' is defined as a set of mental and behavioral steps an individual takes to achieve a specific outcome or goal. Strategies are the processes that underlie your human experience. Many are unconscious and drive our behaviors.

For example, a conscious strategy for problem-solving might involve the following steps:

FIRST: IDENTIFYING THE PROBLEM AND THE DESIRED OUTCOME

Example:

- I am tired all the time, and I want more energy.

SECOND: GATHERING INFORMATION AND ANALYZING THE SITUATION

Example:

- I wake up tired, drink a lot of coffee all day, and then have trouble falling asleep.

- I hate my job.

- I stay up late playing video games.

- I feel tired after eating.

THIRD: GENERATING POSSIBLE SOLUTIONS

Example:

- Drink more caffeine for more energy or other stimulants.

- Eat healthier foods.

- Pick up a drug habit.

- Take sleep medications.

- Exercise

- Get a new job that is more enjoyable.

- Add supplements for energy.

FOURTH: EVALUATING THE SOLUTIONS AND SELECTING THE BEST ONE

Example:

- More coffee and drugs such as cocaine are probably not the best plan.

- More prescription drugs aren't an optimal solution, either.

- Therefore, I will change my diet, take supplements and exercise.

FINALLY: IMPLEMENTING THE SOLUTION AND MONITORING THE RESULTS

Example:

- Change your diet to include healthier foods. Commit to exercise and get a personal trainer. Purchase a supplement protocol and commit to less screen time at night.

NLP emphasizes that strategies can be analyzed and modified to achieve better results. By understanding the mental and behavioral steps involved in achieving a particular outcome, individuals can modify their strategies to become more effective and efficient. I help many clients with this process because, while you probably understand how the above example works, you have unconscious strategies that can sabotage you from making the changes you determined would be beneficial. NLP and hypnosis reprogram the unconscious.

We are all special snowflakes, and this uniqueness extends to our thinking, behavior, and communication. This individuality makes us who we are and is a beautiful aspect of being human. And sometimes we have personal blockages in the form of sabotaging unconscious strategies we constructed as kids to meet our needs. They may hinder personal development, especially in areas such as health and lifestyle, because when we were sad, for example, mom gave us a cookie, and we created a strategy for emotional eating.

This book is not really about anything new. Everyone knows diet, exercise, proper hydration, and sleep benefit health. The secret sauce for creating new habits and making these foundational pieces of health a part of your life is to saddle up your motivation and ride!

There are four primary motivation strategies, and each of us has a unique combination of these strategies that motivates us to take action, and they can show up in different areas of our lives. A 'toward motivation strategy' is when you move toward what you want. For example, you might be motivated to detoxify your body because you want more energy, clearer skin, and better overall health. You can think of this one as a 'carrot' for a horse. The horse is motivated by positive incentives and moves in that direction.

An 'away from motivation strategy' is moving away from what you don't want. For example, you might be motivated to detoxify your body to avoid feeling tired, bloated, and sluggish or from fear of getting a disease associated with toxicity. This is the 'stick.' Horses move away from negative consequences. It is in the same direction inspired by the carrot, but from a different stimulus. Many people are inspired to make lifestyle changes after a scary diagnosis or a heart attack. Wouldn't it be nice to do it before something catastrophic? Before having your ass beat by a stick?

External motivation strategies are triggered by external factors such as rewards, recognition, or pressure from others. Accountability partners are a powerful form of external motivation. Another example is that you might be motivated to detoxify your body because your doctor recommended it or because your friends are also doing it and have encouraged you to join them.

Internally motivated people are inspired by their values and beliefs. For example, you might be motivated to detoxify your body because you believe taking care of your health and well-being is important.

Discipline involves self-control and self-regulation to achieve a desired outcome or goal. It is the ability to consistently act in a certain way or adhere to certain rules or principles, even in the face of difficulties or obstacles.

Discipline helps you deal with your distractions and goals, resist temptation, and persist in facing challenges. It involves setting clear goals, establishing rules and routines, and developing the self-awareness and self-control necessary to act consistently.

The Wilde Life Planner was created to help you be more disciplined. In discipline, you can create new behavior strategies by inspiring neurons to fire together and wire into a new habit. Then, when you come up against obstacles that your old programming wants to quit over, you have new resources and patterns to overcome them.

However, it is important to note that discipline can be overused or misapplied, leading to negative consequences such as burnout or perfectionism.

"Perfectionism is self-abuse of the highest order."
~Anne Wilson Schaef

Balance discipline with self-care, flexibility, and self-compassion to maintain a healthy and sustainable level of motivation. Motivation dancing in tandem with discipline is truly powerful because it combines joy and excitement for what you are doing with processes that lay down new neurology and help to reprogram your behaviors. When your habits become unconscious because you have been disciplined and consistent, you no longer have to continue being 'disciplined.'

By understanding your motivation strategy, you can identify the most likely approach to help you achieve your health and lifestyle goals.

Let's explore how these motivation strategies might apply to you, your health, and your detoxification experience. If one of your major motivation strategies is 'toward,' you are likely to be motivated by the benefits of detoxification. You may find it helpful to focus on the positive outcomes of detoxification, such as increased energy, improved digestion, and clearer skin. You might also find it helpful to set specific goals for your detoxification journey, such as committing to the Wilde Vitality Detoxification Program or giving up sugar for a month.

If your motivation strategy is 'away,' you are likely to be motivated by avoiding the negative consequences of not detoxifying. You may find it helpful to focus on the negative outcomes, such as feeling tired, bloated, and sluggish with more allergies and an increased risk for chronic diseases. You might also find it helpful to set specific consequences for not detoxifying, such as scheduling a doctor's appointment for a full physical and workup if you don't complete your detoxification plan or diverting fun money into a life insurance policy. *Ouch!*

If your primary motivation strategy is internal, you are likely to be motivated by your values and beliefs. So, the following educational part of the book will likely inspire you to make significant health changes and detoxify your whole life. You may, however, find it helpful to reflect on why detoxification is important to you and what it means for your overall health and well-being.

You might also find it helpful to create a daily self-care routine that includes detoxifying practices, such as drinking lemon water in the morning or taking a detoxifying bath in the evening. Chances are you didn't even pick up this book if you are internally motivated because you already have it all in order and scheduled in your high-performance planner.

I created *The Wilde Life Planner* to guide your creation of healthy habits and routines and support your personal growth with Wilde Vitality. The more you use it, the more you will be able to recognize areas where you can improve your habits and optimize your life. Whether you use my planner or another, commit to sitting down each morning and evening to reflect on your process and progress. Accountability and awareness are among the most powerful tools to change your life.

If your main motivation strategy is external, you will likely be motivated by rewards, recognition, or pressure from others. You may find it helpful to enlist the support of others in your detoxification journey, such as an accountability buddy, friend, or family member who is also interested in detoxifying their body. Or you can hire a coach. You might also find setting up a reward system helpful, such as treating yourself to a massage or a new outfit once you complete your detoxification plan. *Yeah!*

Identifying your motivation strategy for improving your health and life is essential to achieving your goals. By understanding your unique combination of motivation strategies, you can tailor your approach to health and better ensure your success because you know how your mind works. I recently recognized that

I have an incredible motivation strategy for 'fixing things' or helping others. By understanding how those strategies worked within me, I was able to transfer them to other areas of my life where I am not so motivated to show up as my best self.

Ask yourself about the last time you were really motivated to do something (nothing was going to stop you) and examine what inspired you.

- What motivates you to pursue your goals?

- What beliefs do you have about your ability to achieve success?

- How do you stay motivated when faced with challenges or setbacks?

- What role does accountability play in your motivation?

- What do you believe are the benefits of achieving your goals?

- What role does your self-talk play in motivating you?

- What do you believe are the consequences of not achieving your goals?

Whew! That was a lot. Give yourself a high five right now for digging through all your old stuff! That took bravery and commitment, and I can tell you are ready to be free of all your old bullshit and committed to creating something new! We have done the inner emotional, mental, and spiritual exploration. Now, let's look at some science about what is going on with your body.

PART II
IT'S COMPLICATED

CHAPTER 6
PHARMOCRACY

Do you feel older than your age, and are you struggling with your health? Do you feel as if health information is overwhelming? Have you tried diet, exercise, medication, and supplements to remedy health concerns you are experiencing, but you don't feel like you got the results you were looking for? Are you stressed out, frustrated, and tired? Are you in pain or feel that weight loss is impossible, no matter how many hours you spend at the gym? Do you feel anxious or depressed? Do you think your hormones are imbalanced, but lab tests returned normal?

Do you feel that conventional medicine doesn't have the answer? Do you feel the desire to be beautiful both inside and out? Do you feel scared of growing older because you can't control your current health experience? You are not alone if you answered 'YES!' to any (or all) of these questions. I will give you three easy-to-understand reasons why you are not feeling well and why what you have done so far hasn't worked.... yet. Then, we explore practical solutions you can apply to your life and see immediate improvements.

You are not alone. Our culture is sick. The younger generations are not expected to live as long as those who have come before. Life expectancy in the U.S. dropped for the second year in a row in 2021. Some demographics within these generations will outlive the others, and what do you think will determine the difference in life spans? Some sources say babies born today will live 150 years, but that is based on extrapolation from history, not reality, and doesn't consider the quality of life. Do you really think AI will save us? I'm not even sure Elon thinks that anymore.

Americans are inundated with pressures to consume, compete, separate from nature, and have shallow, digitized social connections. While cultural pressures and advertisements hypnotize us toward being unhealthy, our medical system has developed into a 'disease management system' rather than a 'health care system.' The healthcare system is the third leading cause of death in the U.S. We have the only for-profit medical system in the developed world, which is also the most expensive and one of the least effective systems for chronic disease.

If you have had a horrible car accident (been there) and need emergency care, you want the U.S. health system. If you have diabetes, heart disease, autoimmunity, allergies, fibromyalgia, cancer, or are pregnant, you want to go anywhere else in the developed world. Insurance companies, pharmaceutical companies, and hospitals are geared more toward profit and managing liability than health.

Let me be very clear. I don't think many individuals go into medicine for fame and fortune. Medicine is a calling, and I believe that providers want what is best for their patients, but their hands are often tied. Hospital conglomerates and HMOs even restrict the research their providers are allowed to read and take into consideration while treating patients.

Providers are strapped with hundreds of thousands of dollars of school debt. They must adhere to what is determined as 'standard of care' based upon policies and procedures to reduce malpractice liability for whatever hospital entity provides their salaried position. Insurance companies dictate what they will pay and how long patients are seen, limiting the amount of time providers can spend. Doctors spend, on average, between 13-19 minutes with each patient. That isn't much time to do an examination, let alone education, and it's just enough time to write a prescription.

Imagine the frustration of being a highly intelligent, powerfully empathetic, and extensively educated medical provider who cannot make the therapeutic decisions you want to make based upon your education and expertise because a group of insurance adjusters, who aren't medically trained, tells you what you can and cannot do. They tell you what is 'medically necessary' based on the financial bottom line, and lawyers! *Ugh.*

The State of California even tried to pass a law prohibiting doctors from giving a medical opinion that differed from what the government party line stated. California tried to label a second opinion 'dangerous disinformation.' British Columbia passed a similar law, stating:

"Non-compliance with Ministry therapeutic guidelines may result in fines up to $200,000 or $500,000 (corporations) and incarceration for up to 6 months. Anonymous complaints to the Ministry regarding a practitioner can be publicized, and the practitioner's license suspended before investigation. Ministry agents may now enter a healthcare practice, seize patient charts, and restrict access to that facility without notice or court order."

No wonder physician suicide is among the highest in any profession.

Insurance reimbursement also determines which laboratory analyses and imaging studies are allowed. Often, the least expensive, bare-minimum labs are run, so the clues to why you aren't feeling well are entirely missed until the problem becomes so big it can no longer be ignored.

The labs most often performed at a yearly physical are a complete blood count (CBC) with differential and a comprehensive metabolic panel (CMP). These labs will tell you if you have anemia, blood cancer, or liver or kidney failure. If you complain of fatigue, you may have Thyroid Stimulating Hormone (TSH) ordered, and if it is age-appropriate, a lipid panel will check your cholesterol.

If you pay cash for those labs, they cost under $50. If insurance is billed, they will likely pay between $150 and $200. Most health problems you are concerned about will not be addressed or diagnosed by these labs. Lab ranges are designed for 90% of the population and are certainly not geared toward optimization. Screening tests like TSH are grossly inaccurate. Running TSH to understand how the thyroid functioning is like someone asking your grandmother about your sex life. It is two full generations away from what we want to know.

But insurance will often pay for TSH, and no further thyroid tests will be run if it is in the 'normal range.' The ranges of conventional lab work are designed to only look for gross dysfunction rather than imbalances that can be rectified to optimize health. The average range for TSH labs is 0.45 to 4.5 mIU/L. I know a person's thyroid is struggling if their TSH is over 2 mIU/L, and I implement strategies to help it work better.

To add insult to injury, conventional care does almost nothing for prevention. Their top recommendations for 'prevention' are screening tests or taking a baby aspirin every day. That isn't prevention; that's medication and early detection. The pharmaceutical industry has the largest lobby in Washington, D.C., with 1,834 registered lobbyists. That equals more than 3 lobbyists for each representative. When I started writing this book a few years ago, there were only 1,200. Top pharmaceutical companies spend millions of dollars to manipulate research, control product consumption, and masterfully market and create diseases to fit the drugs they are researching. Most drugs are expensive Band-Aids; they don't address the cause of disease, and they merely manage symptoms to the tune of $1.48 trillion in revenue in 2022.

It is a brilliant business model, creating perpetual consumers who never expected to get better. The markup on medications is astronomical. For example, the cost to cure Hepatitis C in the U.S. is between $39,000 and $94,000 for the 12-week course of medication. In India, where the medications are manufactured, the cost for the full course of treatment is $900. That is a 4300% markup and a lot of profit.

"For the love of money is the root of all evil."
~Timothy 6:10, King James Bible

Modern medicine is riding on the merits of the 1928 discovery of antibiotics and has become a drug culture. To be fair, antibiotics and antivirals do treat the causes of many diseases they are prescribed for. Still, over-prescribing antibiotics creates 'superbugs' like MRSA and dangerous diseases like C. diff diarrhea and other gastrointestinal diseases. A recent seven-year-long study found that chronic antibiotic use in middle-aged women was linked to mild cognitive decline. Antibiotic use also increases the risk of Inflammatory Bowel Diseases (IBD), Ulcerative Colitis, and Crohn's disease. I attended Naturopathic Medical School to explore wellness and disease prevention in an attempt to ease humanity's suffering. I have a DEA number and can prescribe medications if necessary, but I usually choose not to. I taught pharmacology for a Nurse Practitioner program, and I understand how drugs work and when it is best to prescribe them. Most often, I choose herbal medicine, vitamins, minerals, and other natural substances recognized and processed like food in the body. When used correctly, they do not have side effects. They help people heal rather than cover up symptoms of the disease.

There is a time and a place for prescription drugs, but there is a spectrum of progression between when you can first see the evidence of disease if you know how and where to look and when a drug prescription becomes necessary for the rest of someone's life. That is why I chose to be a naturopathic physician—to practice true prevention and health care. The sooner you address the cause of the disease you are creating, the easier it is to reverse it. Please don't wait until it is too late and you have a heart attack, develop an autoimmune disease, or are diagnosed with late-stage cancer. Do something now to improve your health and quality of life for the long term. That is your best health insurance.

Think about how much you pay for medical care. Then, think about how you are never expected to get better if the disease you have isn't an infection. I have helped clients experience a reversal of their symptoms and disease more times than I can tell you, and their primary care professional very rarely asked them how they did it. I think that is borderline criminal. If you saw cervical dysplasia reversed naturally without a dangerous procedure that could make a patient unable to have children, wouldn't you want to know how it was done? For many drugs, once you are prescribed to be on them, you are expected to continue for the rest of your life.

More medications will then be prescribed to manage the side effects of the first prescriptions. Pharmacists will tell you that once three prescriptions are in the body, there is no way to predict the possible side effects that will be seen because the chemistry is too complex.

I saw a commercial recently for *Tardive Dyskinesia*, or 'T.D.' T.D. is a movement disorder with uncontrollable, abnormal, repetitive neurological tics, commonly eye, mouth, tongue, or cheek movements. The only way you get T.D. is as a side effect of another drug, usually from antipsychotics. You don't get T.D. any other way. This is the first prescription medication I know of that was developed entirely to manage the side effects of another. It may alarm you further that antipsychotic medications are often used for 'treatment-resistant' anxiety and depression.

> *"If your only tool is a hammer, then every problem looks like a nail."*
> **~Abraham Maslow**

Conventional medicine prescribes one drug to manage a symptom, often creating a side effect that triggers a prescribing cascade of other drugs to treat the side effects. Consider this possible prescription cascade:

As a baby, you have acid reflux. Often this comes from a food sensitivity to something your mother is eating or the chemical soy, wheat, corn, dairy, artificial, and toxic shitshow that is baby formula. No one in conventional care educates your mother about how to make lifestyle changes to help you. Instead, you are prescribed a proton pump inhibitor (PPI), esomeprazole, or Nexium, which is FDA-approved for patients younger than one year.

This immediately compromises your body's ability to digest food properly, decreasing the absorption of vitamins, minerals, and proteins. Common side effects include headaches, nausea, diarrhea, gas, constipation, dry mouth, and drowsiness. Most notably, it inhibits the absorption of B12, a vitally important vitamin for brain and nerve health. PPI medications are associated with H. pylori, gastric cancers, celiac disease, C. diff infections, and dementia. You are also likely low in calcium and magnesium. Magnesium is necessary for more than 300 biochemical reactions in the body. You probably know calcium is needed to keep your bones strong, and it also plays a role in your nerve and brain function, every beat of your heart, and every single muscle contraction you make.

Taking a PPI causes you to grow up with a compromised gut due to an imbalanced microbiome and decreased digestive secretions, leading to leaky gut, inflammation, and worsening food sensitivities. Decreasing stomach acid has been connected with seasonal allergies, but don't worry; you can take Claritin, or loratadine, every day for that. Mild side effects include headaches, drowsiness, fatigue, nervousness, stomach pain, and diarrhea. Food sensitivities are also associated with eczema and atopy, including asthma. So, you are given topical cortisone and an inhaler.

You now have trouble paying attention in school with all the inflammation, fatigue, headaches, and nutrient deficiencies. Your parents love you and want to help you succeed in school, but they aren't given any other options to support your learning, and you are prescribed Adderall: amphetamine/dextroamphetamine mixed salts. Yes, you read that correctly: amphetamine. Common side effects of Adderall are loss of appetite, weight loss, stomach upset and pain, dizziness, nervousness, trouble sleeping, and increased blood sugar that sets you up to develop diabetes. Your inhaler also leads to anxiety and sleep disturbances. You know sleep is essential, so to counteract the difficulty sleeping, you are prescribed Ambien, which is associated with the same cancer risk as smoking if you take it more than 17 times a year. Not just Ambien, but anything that drugs your brain to sleep, be it alcohol, Benadryl, etc., increases your risk of cancer significantly. Conventional medicine doesn't know why there is an association; I think it is because your cortisol is high at night from stress.

Cortisol shuts off the immune system, so when you shut your brain off to get some sleep, the cortisol stays high because you haven't addressed the problem. One of the jobs of your immune system is to go around your body at night and find cancer cells, kill them, and do other repairs. If it is suppressed by cortisol, it isn't doing that.

And you still aren't getting good enough regenerative sleep. You feel stressed and depressed because, along with 'nervousness,' a euphemism for anxiety, other Adderall side effects include weakness, constipation, less interest in sex, difficulty keeping an erection, elevated blood pressure, and twitching. You may be headed down the pathway to being prescribed medication for your depression, which will likely further impact your sex life and also increase the likelihood you will develop metabolic syndrome and diabetes due to the associated weight gain.

In early 2023, a study came out showing that diabetes patients taking a PPI (remember the drug you were put on as a baby?) had a 27% higher chance of developing coronary artery disease, a 34% higher risk of heart attack, a 35% higher risk of heart failure, and a 30% higher increase in the risk of death from all causes.

So, you are put on a blood pressure medication that makes you tired and impairs your ability to have sex. Your cholesterol is high, and now you are given a statin drug associated with dementia risk and heart failure.

What a clusterfuck. Even writing about it makes me angry. And scenarios like that happen daily to people who don't look outside the conventional system.

Here's a message from my lawyers: Ask your doctor if being on an average of five medications after age 40 is right for you.

No, wait... that was a big pharma ad. And there is only one other country in the world that allows drug Ads on television.

Hmm.

Here's the AI generated disclaimer from my lawyers:

"The information provided in this book is for general informational purposes only and is not intended to be a substitute for professional medical advice, diagnosis, or treatment. Always seek the advice of your physician or other qualified health provider with any questions you may have regarding a medical condition.

The author and publisher of this book have made reasonable efforts to ensure that the information provided is accurate and up to date at the time of publication, or at least in agreement with the fascist government agenda, so we are not suspiciously murdered or commit suicide. However, they make no representations or warranties of any kind, express or implied, about the completeness, accuracy, reliability, suitability, or availability concerning the information contained within this book.

In all seriousness, I don't recommend completely ignoring the benefits of pharmaceutical drugs and life-saving surgical procedures when necessary, and I am alive because of them. However, there is a considerable amount of time between the first symptoms or indications of a disease and its worsening to the point where medication and surgery are your only options.

And remember, conventional providers can either not give integrative, alternative, and lifestyle advice because their associations don't let them, and they can be legitimately attacked and their medical license threatened, or they are only trained in drugs and surgery and conventional nutritional advice that brings us the steaming pile of dog shit we call 'hospital food.' Beware the provider that tells you that 'diet doesn't matter' and get a different one. A recent projection predicted that over a billion people will have diabetes by 2050; the good news is that it can be reversed with diet.

I hope this book helps you realize where you stand with your health and gives you the resources needed to identify where your body isn't working optimally. You can then change your lifestyle to reverse the disease processes before needing medications for the rest of your life and well before undergoing surgeries that may or may not successfully eradicate your symptoms. Did you know that more than 40% of gallbladder surgeries don't resolve abdominal pain, and once your gallbladder is out, you won't properly digest your fats and fat-soluble vitamins without support. Not absorbing healthy fats sets you up for inflammation and neurological problems. Wouldn't you rather be proactive?

Thanks to antibiotics, chronic diseases are one of the leading health issues in the developing world. Two centuries ago, people were much more likely to die of infection than diabetes (unless you were an indolent royal and ate a lot of cake like Marie Antoinette and her BFFs). The most recent "golden age" of medicine began with the discovery of penicillin and other antibiotics, which saved more lives than anything else in history and then promptly became part of the problem.

When we talk about 'treating the cause of disease' and not the symptoms, antimicrobials, antivirals, and antifungals treat part of the cause because they kill the overgrowth of organisms causing the problem. Antibiotics can save lives because the immune system cannot always mount a sufficient attack against invaders. Unfortunately, over-prescribing antimicrobials for diseases that aren't caused by bacteria (most ear infections in children are viral) has created a HUGE problem, leading to superbugs. You've no doubt heard of MRSA—Methicillin-Resistant Staph Aureus.

Additionally, the medical establishment decided pills were the way to go. I support researching the history of American medicine more deeply if you want to head down the rabbit hole. I won't speak much to it here except to say it is a brilliant business model that never solves the problem, creates increased dependency, and ensures return business. The medical industry is now the most powerful lobby in the U.S., funneling billions to legislators and government agencies like the CDC and FDA. They fund every conventional medical school and have successfully created a system that only prescribes drugs and surgery for every ailment and ostracizes or suppresses anything that deviates from their party line, no matter what the science says.

Medicine is a practice, and everyone is different. Research and statistics can be skewed to support a chosen agenda. Conventional providers can't be expected to know everything. You are responsible for exploring options and educating yourself to make the most informed health decisions for yourself and your family.

Drugs and surgery are the best options for people who do not want to make changes to their lifestyles. Many people just want to take a pill and get on with their lives. Others have the bejeezus scared out of them with outdated research or are shamed into doing what their provider recommends. I am not one of those people, and if you aren't either, these resources will guide you on your health adventure to make healthy choices from an informed position of power rather than fear.

CHAPTER 7
THE POWER OF LIFESTYLE

There are three major components to developing disease in your body, and we encounter them constantly as we navigate modern life. They feed on one another, and unless they are all adequately addressed, your health concerns will likely remain an issue for you.

These components are Stress, Inflammation, and Toxicity. Let's look at where you encounter these during a typical day.

WHAT DO YOU DO EVERYDAY?

Wake up tired: Not getting enough regenerative sleep is terrible for everything in your body (stress).

- **Shower**: Exposed to toxicants in water, body wash, soap, shampoo, conditioner, shaving cream, etc.

- **Brush teeth**: Exposed to toxicants in toothpaste, dental floss, and mouthwash. The thin skin of your mouth is a great absorptive surface, which is why some medications are prescribed to be dissolved under the tongue for quick action.

- **Do hair and makeup**: Exposed to toxicants in makeup, perfume, hair products, antiperspirants, moisturizers, etc.

- **Get dressed:** Exposure to detergents, dryer sheets, and dry-cleaning toxicants. Microfibers and synthetic fabrics also add to microplastic pollution in the world.

- **Eat breakfast**: Whatever is easy and compliments coffee. Usually carbohydrate heavy foods like cereal, granola, bagels, toast, muffins, English muffins, which are then paired with dairy – frosting, cream cheese, cream, and milk.

The spikes in your blood sugar from too many carbs in the morning can quickly leave you in a slump, craving candy and more carbs. Grains and dairy are famously inflammatory for most people, leading to digestive problems, acne, pain, hormone imbalances, fatigue, allergies, and the inability to lose weight. More on this later.

- **Commute to work in traffic**: Air pollution around highways has been tied to chronic disease and neurological problems. Air pollution has been proven to make diabetes worse.

- **Work all day at a job that doesn't make your heart sing:** Do you want to go through your whole life working a job that doesn't inspire you, feeling underappreciated, underpaid, underutilized, and all-around MEH?

- **Stress at work**: What do you think stress does to your health and well-being? I'll give you a hint... it is not good.

- **Sit at work**: Sedentary behavior increases all-cause mortality, cardiovascular disease mortality, cancer risk, and risks of metabolic disorders such as diabetes, high blood pressure, and high cholesterol. It leads to pain and osteoporosis, depression and dementia. This is all well supported by conventional medical literature.

- **Make poor food choices for lunch**: Do you eat junk food, fast food or microwave a premade meal in the microwave? Do you go out to eat and consume 1450 calories from Cheesecake Factory's Cobb Salad?

- **Commute home in traffic**: Again, more toxicants and more stress.

- **Make/eat dinner**: The choices we make about food play a HUGE role in how we feel daily and the diseases we are at risk for. If you eat toxic and pro-inflammatory foods, your body will not thrive and repair itself.

- **Do chores, errands, housework, pay bills, walk the dog, etc:** This can be stressful, especially if we are overtired, overscheduled, or overwhelmed.

- **Unwind:** Watching TV, social media interaction, or online gaming.

Did you know the more exposure to media you have, the more your self-esteem and mood plummet? Your stress increases due to fear-mongering, bad news, and violence on every channel.

Additionally, you are exposed to light and stimulus, making it difficult for your brain to shut down properly and get the deep, restful sleep essential to optimal body functioning.

- **Going out:** Going out and drinking your woes away slowly poisons your body.

- **Dating:** App dating can be a long line of casual hookups or disappointing dates without a real human connection.

- **Go to sleep and hope it is a restful night:** Then you wake up, rinse, and repeat. All the while, you keep dreaming about the weekend and counting the days until vacation.

If you're reading this and thinking, "*WTF, every aspect of my life erodes my health and well-being! It is time to stop the insanity!*" This book is for you!

Health is complicated because our modern society is assaulting it from every direction. The air, water, food, personal care products, social interactions, fear-mongering media, cultural expectations, radiation, pollution, etc., all detract from your vitality.

Don't lose your mind, even though there is poison everywhere you look. There is hope. When I learn new horrifying facts like flame retardants in baby pajamas are absorbed through the skin, are extremely toxic and capable of causing disease, I remind myself of the serenity prayer.

I altered it a little to serve my purpose:

Grant me the serenity to accept the things I cannot change. (We swim in a chemical soup of toxicity.)

The courage to change the things I can. (What I eat, drink, breathe, buy, and how I choose to behave.)

And the wisdom to know the difference.

I wrote this book to help you understand "the difference" and have the courage to change what you can. I wrote it to empower you to regain control over your health through lifestyle and making educated choices about how you live 80–90% of the time. This method will allow you to stay up late, drink too much wine, and have fun sometimes without torpedoing your health. For example, you can't do much about toxic air on your commute. You can insulate your body and decrease exposure by getting air filters for your house.

You will get information here in a holistic way and actionable items to incorporate into your life through micro-movements. This is the best investment you can make in yourself, your body, your long-term health, and your life.

CHAPTER 8
STRESS

Even before 2020, Americans had increasing stress and decreased resources to manage it. Over time, heightened stress levels ultimately lead to significant changes in your health status by impacting your mental, cardiovascular, metabolic, immune, hormonal, and digestive health.

Do you remember the last time you felt really stressed? I bet your heart was racing, your face and head felt hot from the rise in blood pressure, your palms probably started sweating, and your stomach may have felt upset.

When stressed, your autonomic (automatic) nervous system switches to favor sympathetic output, preparing your body to fight, flee, or freeze. Before the modern era, human lives were much more difficult; danger was everywhere, and many had to physically fight to survive. To optimize survival, the sympathetic system increases heart rate, shunts blood to the muscles, deepens the rate and depth of breathing for oxygen supply, increases fuel in the blood (blood sugar), and dilates the eyes. This response is great when you have to fight a bear.

It isn't so great when it happens in traffic and never really stops because of our high-paced, demanding modern lives. Unfortunately, the human brain can't differentiate between situations that threaten our lives and situations that threaten us in our jobs, relationships, and finances—those that threaten our livelihood, security, ego, and status quo.

The main stress hormone is cortisol, which increases the risk of heart disease, stroke, and other health problems. Stress can also weaken the immune system, making the body more susceptible to infections and illnesses. Mentally, stress can contribute to depression, anxiety, and sleep disturbances and interfere with cognitive functioning and memory. In addition, chronic stress can lead to muscle tension, headaches, and digestive issues such as irritable bowel syndrome.

Stress has been shown to disrupt the balance of sex hormones in both men and women. Stress can lower testosterone levels in men, leading to decreased sexual desire and performance. In women, stress can disrupt the menstrual cycle, cause irregular periods, and lead to infertility.

Cortisol also affects the functioning of the Hypothalamic-pituitary thyroid (HPT) axis, which regulates the production and release of thyroid hormones. Thyroid hormones, such as triiodothyronine (T3) and thyroxine (T4), are critical in regulating the body's metabolism.

Thyroid hormones stimulate the conversion of food into energy and affect the rate at which cells use energy. Elevated cortisol levels, as seen during chronic stress, can suppress the HPT axis and lead to decreased thyroid hormone production, resulting in hypothyroidism symptoms, including fatigue, weight gain, and depression.

Cortisol also impacts insulin sensitivity and glucose metabolism, leading to elevated blood sugar levels and an increased risk of developing insulin resistance and type 2 diabetes. When I see TSH over 2, I know the adrenal glands need support.

Cortisol and epinephrine are two hormones released in response to stress and play a role in mental health and regulating emotions. Epinephrine, also known as adrenaline, is a catecholamine hormone produced by the adrenal medulla. Both cortisol and epinephrine can significantly impact mental health and the regulation of emotions, including anxiety and depression, because they impact neurotransmitter levels in the brain.

Cortisol has been shown to decrease neurotransmitters such as serotonin and dopamine, which regulate mood. At the same time, epinephrine increases the levels of norepinephrine, which is associated with increased vigilance and anxiety. Chronic exposure to high levels of cortisol and epinephrine, as seen during chronic stress, can lead to long-term changes in the regulation of neurotransmitters and contribute to the development of anxiety and depression.

You may have heard that life is 10% what happens to you and 90% how you respond. This is largely accurate, yet if you are already overwhelmed and stressed out and experiencing the downstream effects listed above, you are more likely to respond poorly to something going sideways in your life.

The average American is overscheduled in day-to-day routines and overstressed due to the pressures of life and societal expectations; pandemics, the threat of world war, and inflation only worsen it. If you were stressed out by the theoretical schedule above, imagine how it becomes even more hectic and unmanageable when you add a spouse, children, and other responsibilities. Many professionals tend to neglect their health and put self-care off until *"sometime after"* or *"when I have enough ...."*

The best way to manage stress is to allow yourself to rest and be gentle with yourself. The other side of the autonomic (automatic) nervous system is the parasympathetic system, which supports rest, digestion, and repair. That is why we spent time identifying your unhealthy patterns and where you spend time that does not serve you. When you understand your default programming and know where to make and schedule changes, you can instill self-care into your patterning.

Taking "a moment" is so much more powerful than taking a chill pill. Making yourself a priority and enjoying life's little luxuries is a constructive way to 'treat yourself' because it fundamentally heals stress. I hope you are inspired to manage your stress, decreasing the chances of developing chronic diseases such as cardiovascular disease, diabetes, cancer, autoimmunity, digestive disorders, depression, infertility, and anxiety.

If you already suffer from one or more of these ailments, stress management will help you slow their progression and may even reverse them.

NLP practitioners often use a technique called 'tasking.' We assign a negative consequence—something the client, under no circumstances, wants to happen. The aversion to the consequence provides 'away from' motivation to prioritize and complete the assigned tasks. Completing the 'tasking' creates new neurology; it connects your brain cells into new pathways, a different way of behaving is born, and a habit is created.

When I went through my training, if I did not keep my agreements, my consequence was to tell one of my brothers that I was undisciplined and had wasted thousands of dollars on something. Even thinking of doing that caused my body to heat up, and there was NO WAY I would let that happen. I committed to the process and completed the task before me; it was great motivation! Committing to a consequence is something we often do unconsciously. If you drink too much, you get a hangover. If you run a red light in front of a cop, you get a ticket. Committing to a consequence for not showing up for ourselves isn't something many of us do. When we break resolutions and don't prioritize ourselves, the consequences aren't immediate. They exist somewhere in the nebulous future when we develop diabetes, have a stroke, or get cancer.

That is another reason why accountability processes and partners support your success, external motivation, and adherence to our agreed commitment.

What new behaviors will you create in response to stress? Instead of emotionally eating, will you walk outside instead? Who will hold you accountable? What will be the consequences of not showing up for yourself when you need them to be? It may serve to contemplate whether you would show up for a friend in need. If so, why don't you show up for yourself? What is holding you back from valuing, loving, and caring for yourself?

No matter how you want to explain how screens and technology can relax you, that is not the case. Break free from your digital overlords and choose activities that are not on a screen or centered around alcohol and food. Choose something outside with someone you love, like a brother, a friend or a dog.

SCREEN-LESS, SOBER STRESS-BUSTING ACTIVITY EXAMPLES INCLUDE:

- Meditation and deep breathing exercises.

- Journaling and creative writing.
- Exercise, such as yoga, running, or weightlifting.
- Art therapy, such as painting or drawing.
- Gardening and spending time in nature.
- Hobbies such as knitting, woodworking, or playing an instrument.
- Reading a book or listening to an audiobook.
- Cooking or baking.
- Volunteering or helping others.
- Playing games, such as board games or card games.
- Taking a walk or going for a hike.
- Practicing mindfulness and gratitude.
- Learning a new skill, such as a language or musical instrument.
- Massage or self-care activities.
- Getting a pet and spending time with them.
- Taking a bath or relaxing in a hot tub.
- Spending quality time with loved ones.
- Practicing relaxation techniques, such as progressive muscle relaxation.
- Doing a puzzle or crossword.
- Taking a nap or getting a good night's sleep.

What are you committed to doing to help you manage your stress?

CHAPTER 9
INFLAMMATION

The human body is miraculous. It can heal itself, which is an absolute miracle if you take the time to think about it. Like stress, inflammation is a normal, healthy, and necessary part of life. Chronic stress has catastrophic effects on the body, and the same goes for chronic, rampant inflammation.

Healthy inflammation is a natural response of the body to injury or infection. The immune system activates and sends white blood cells and signaling chemicals to the site of injury or infection to repair damage and fight off the harmful agent. This process is known as acute inflammation and is a normal and necessary part of healing. However, chronic stress can lead to persistent low-grade inflammation, which harms the body. You read above that cortisol has many actions in the body; it also helps to regulate the immune system.

When cortisol levels are elevated, part of the immune system becomes suppressed, and the body is less able to fight off infections and heal from injuries. Sustained activation of the stress response system has also been shown to increase the production and release of pro-inflammatory cytokines, which are proteins that promote unhealthy inflammation. When levels of these cytokines are elevated due to chronic stress, they can contribute to various health problems, such as cardiovascular disease, depression, digestive issues, autoimmunity, and other stress-related disorders.

HOW IS THIS SYSTEM ACTIVATED?

A healthy immune system learns the difference between 'self' and 'not-self' during infancy. The immune system is programmed to respond to foreign proteins that are not 'self.' Usually, these proteins are bacteria, fungi, or viruses. That is partly why little kids are sick all the time, their immune system is learning how to protect the body from invasion. This is also the premise of vaccination. Teaching the immune system how to respond to specific diseases.

Autoimmunity is when the immune system can no longer differentiate between foreign proteins and proteins that belong to the body or 'self.' In autoimmune diseases like Lupus, the immune system attacks and damages blood vessels, while in rheumatoid arthritis, joints are the recipients of the inappropriate immune response.

Just about every disease has an element of inflammation, which makes sense because the body is trying to heal itself. Diabetes, heart disease, inability to lose weight, insomnia, fatigue, cancer, anxiety, depression, eczema, psoriasis, asthma, thyroid issues, hair loss, aging, pain, and mental disorders are all worsened by rampant inflammation.

Inflammation is like a slow-burning fire inside the body, causing damage and disease. How can the harmful inflammation be turned down and extinguished? You need to first eliminate what is causing the problem. Otherwise, it is like throwing gasoline on fire at the same time you are trying to put it out. One of my first explorations with every client is determining which foods increase inflammation in the body.

Avoiding food sensitivities is something that can be

done every day to decrease inflammation. I don't run IgG or IgM testing for foods; those are what you can get through your regular doctor. I don't find them as accurate as the cell-mediated tests, which take out your white blood cells, culture them, and then expose them to food proteins and watch how much they freak out by releasing histamine and cytokines. It is a functional test approximating what is happening in your own body.

WHY NOT USE ANTI-INFLAMMATORY DRUGS?

Non-steroidal anti-inflammatory drugs (NSAIDs), like naproxen, ibuprofen, and aspirin, can be taken to temporarily alleviate the pain caused by inflammation by blocking enzymes that contribute to inflammation. They are beneficial for heinous hangovers and other special occasions. Next-level anti-inflammatory drug options include prednisone and cortisone. Prednisone is a life-saving medication for when you have to suppress the immune system because if you don't, it could kill you, like in severe autoimmune diseases and life-threatening asthma.

Cortisone injections are often used in joints to decrease pain when pain relievers are no longer strong enough. Using both of these drugs mimics the effects of cortisol, which you read about earlier, and avoiding them helps reduce stress on the body. As I have said, there is a time and place for medication, and prednisone does save lives. You don't want to use it long-term, so addressing the cause of the inflammation supports your long-term success.

While pain and inflammatory symptoms can be managed for a while with medications, there are always side effects. NSAIDs can cause stomach pain and ulcers, an increased risk of heart attack and stroke, allergic reactions, liver and kidney problems, headaches, dizziness, and a tendency to bleed more. Long-term use can also increase your risk of kidney, breast, and endometrial cancer. Immunomodulators are drugs prescribed for autoimmune diseases, and one of their most common side effects is cancer. The immune system constantly scours your body for cancer cells; if you suppress that function, your cancer risk skyrockets.

Acetaminophen, or Tylenol, has been shown to change how the brain reacts to emotions, suppressing empathy, and it can cause liver damage. The most significant class action lawsuit in history (to date—just wait for the one against plastic) has named acetaminophen (generic Tylenol) as a cause of autism. Women taking Tylenol during pregnancy were shown to have a statistically significant increased risk of having a baby with autism.

Prednisone and other corticosteroids cause abdominal weight gain, anxiety, a fat face, a buffalo hump (I am not kidding—it's fat on the base of your neck), and fatigue. Cortisone shots make joints weaker and more damaged over time, and they may affect your other hormones.

Some health experts may argue that you need to avoid all unhealthy, inflammatory substances like alcohol, fried food, etc., all the time and eat like a saint. However, sucking the fun out of life sounds terrible to me! I am a proponent of education, moderation, and mindset reprogramming. By making significant dietary changes for a few months, healing your leaky gut, and supporting your body in other ways, you will have significantly improved your health and can return to enjoying your favorite foods in moderation without dire consequences. Don't be surprised if they don't taste the same or if you recognize that they make you feel ill. Those are the connections we want you to make. Get in touch with your body to make informed decisions about whether those nasty, fake supermarket cupcakes are worth eating or whether you are eating your emotions, acting out one of your mother's patterns, and/or experiencing an addiction.

HAVE YOU HEARD OF LEAKY GUT?

In our culture of consumerism and drive to succeed, we often neglect our bodies for years in the name of work, social status, responsibilities, and other pressures. We lose touch with what makes us feel healthy because we stop paying attention. How often have you eaten something and later felt sick to your stomach? But you eat it anyway? That food is causing inflammation and eroding your health.

Stress and inflammation combine to create intestinal permeability, also known as 'Leaky Gut.' It is a condition in which the gut barrier becomes more permeable, allowing substances such as undigested food particles and harmful bacteria to leak into the bloodstream and lead to inflammation. Remember how the immune system is supposed to attack foreign proteins? This is precisely what happens, and it leads to the release of pro-inflammatory cytokines and immune signaling molecules, otherwise known as 'throwing gasoline on the fire,' leading to autoimmune diseases and other health problems.

Stress is one of the leading causes of a leaky gut. Chronic stress leads to the release of cortisol, and the body behaves more in the sympathetic "fight, flight or freeze" behaviors. The parasympathetic system regulates rest, digestion, and repair, so digestion is shut down when the body is in a stressful state. This leads to food proteins not being wholly digested and broken down into amino acids, and the gut lining not being maintained and repaired adequately. Additionally, stress can cause constipation and changes in the gut microbiome, which is the collection of microorganisms that live in the gut. These changes can lead to an overgrowth of harmful bacteria and a decrease in beneficial bacteria, further contributing to a leaky gut.

Food sensitivities occur when the immune system reacts to certain foods, leading to symptoms such as bloating, abdominal pain, chronic pain, allergies, weight gain, fatigue, autoimmunity, IBS etc. Foods commonly associated with food sensitivities include gluten, dairy, soy, nightshades, citrus, and artificial sweeteners. However, food sensitivities vary widely from person to person and are often related to the things most frequently consumed.

THE IMPACT OF AVOIDING INFLAMMATORY FOODS

I graduated from Cornell in a wheelchair because I almost lost my leg in a car accident my senior year. First responders didn't think anyone could be alive in the car and used the jaws of life to get us out. They saved my life, and the surgeon saved my leg. I don't have any physical impairments or restrictions, and I can downhill ski, run, and backpack despite being bedridden for months and told I would be lucky if I even walked again.

Some life events divide your lifetime into 'before' and 'after.' After that car accident, I was invigorated with incredible gratitude to be alive and recognized that I could have died at 21, and every day was, in fact, a gift. I was also given the choice to lie down and feel sorry for myself or fight for my life. I fought. In my early thirties, however, I took Vicodin and Valium to sleep some nights because the pain was unbearable. I couldn't face the rest of my life being in that much pain and I started exploring other options. Up to that point, I had done physical therapy, yoga, massage, chiropractic, acupuncture, reiki, craniosacral therapy, and prolotherapy. All those avenues helped, but I was still in severe pain.

I thought about what I would do for one of my patients with intractable pain, and finally did a food sensitivity panel on myself. It was low on my list because I didn't recognize any digestive issues at the time. The report revealed that I was sensitive to coffee, chocolate, cauliflower, coconut, and turkey, just to name a few. Do you know how turkey is supposed to be so healthy? I was eating it almost every day.

After throwing a mini hissy fit about how the test couldn't possibly be right and there was no way I was giving up chocolate and coffee, I did an elimination diet and avoided those major sensitivities for six months. I repaired my gut and allowed my immune system to reset. Most of the foods no longer bother me, but I haven't been able to eat turkey for years. I also haven't had to take Vicodin or Valium. On Thanksgiving, I have a grass-fed ribeye rather than turkey because, no matter how delicious it may be, it isn't worth feeling like I got hit by a bus for three days.

These are the connections that I hope you make for yourself. What is raising your inflammation? Connect what you are eating with how you feel. It saved my life, and it can save yours.

CHAPTER 10
TOXICITY

In 2017, the World Health Organization (WHO) released a report stating that pollution caused the deaths of more people than all the war and violence on the planet combined. Pollution is harmful because it contains 'toxicants' that damage and poison the human body. Toxicants, also known as toxic substances, toxins or chemicals, are substances that can cause harm to living organisms, including humans, and are known to cause chronic disease. Chemical exposure is a common source of toxicants and can come from various sources, such as the air we breathe, the food we eat, and the products we use daily.

I've been researching and practicing environmental medicine for 20 years and recognize the role of environmental chemicals in human disease. Chemical exposure has been linked to various health problems, including cancer, congenital disabilities, developmental disorders, neurological problems, and reproductive problems. Some chemicals, such as lead, mercury, benzene, Volatile organic compounds (VOCs), plasticizers, and pesticides, have been shown to have particularly harmful effects on human health.

Toxic exposures result in oxidative stress, an imbalance between the production of free radicals and the body's ability to neutralize them. Free radicals are highly reactive molecules that can damage cells and contribute to the development of chronic diseases such as heart disease, cancer, and neurological disorders. Have you heard of antioxidants? They are beneficial because they reverse oxidative stress.

The impact of chemical exposure on human health can vary depending on several factors, including the type of chemical, the duration and frequency of exposure, the age and health of the individual, and genetic factors. Some individuals may be more susceptible to the harmful effects of chemical exposure due to their genetic makeup and how well they can remove the chemicals from their bodies. Children are especially vulnerable due to their smaller size and developing bodies.

Do you experience any of the following?

- Fatigue
- Allergies
- Depression
- Postnasal drip
- Chronic Infections
- Headaches and migraines
- Joint pain and muscle aches
- Gas and bloating
- Insomnia
- Infertility and PCOS
- Rashes
- Eczema
- Psoriasis
- Acne
- Bloating
- PMS

- Irregular and/or painful periods
- Infertility
- Hair Loss
- Brain fog and memory issues
- Anxiety
- Cancer
- Autoimmunity
- Sensitivity to chemical smells like perfumes, gasoline, tires
- Difficulty losing weight
- Vertigo
- Tinnitus
- Memory issues
- Type II Diabetes
- High Cholesterol
- Thyroid disease
- Chronic Fatigue or Fibromyalgia

If you answered 'yes' to any of the above, environmental toxicity is likely a significant cause of your health concerns. If you live on Earth, toxicity is likely a significant cause of your health concerns, and continued exposure will only worsen your health, speed up your aging, and increase your mortality. Environmental Medicine practitioners often say, *"Genetics points the gun, and toxicity pulls the trigger."*

COMMON TOXINS

Mycotoxins are substances that are produced by certain fungi and can have a detrimental impact on human health. These toxic substances can contaminate various food and water sources and are responsible for various illnesses and health issues in humans. I often test my most complicated patient cases to determine if they have been exposed to mycotoxins.

Water damage in a building creates an ideal environment for fungi to grow and multiply. The presence of moisture and organic materials provides the perfect breeding ground for various types of fungi, including those that produce mycotoxins. When these toxins are present in the environment, they can contaminate the air and water sources, leading to significant health risks for those exposed.

Aflatoxin is one of the most well-known mycotoxins. This toxin is known to cause liver damage and can even increase the risk of liver cancer. It is commonly found in peanuts. Other types of mycotoxins, such as ochratoxin and trichothecenes, can also harm human health by impacting the immune system, causing kidney damage, and neurological effects.

The symptoms of mycotoxin exposure can vary depending on the individual and the type of toxin present. Respiratory problems, skin irritation, and allergic reactions are common symptoms of mycotoxin exposure. People with pre-existing respiratory conditions, such as asthma, may be particularly vulnerable to the effects of mycotoxins. Long-term exposure to mycotoxins has also been linked to various health problems, including headaches, fatigue, and neurological symptoms.

When water damage occurs in a building, it is critical to clean up the water and repair any damage as quickly as possible to prevent the growth of fungi. Get a top-of-the-line air purifier to remove spores and maintain indoor air quality. You want a professional to assist you with any mold damage because you want it done correctly to ensure the mold is completely eradicated.

Mold has been a significant health concern since the Old Testament days; Leviticus has a whole section about how to deal with mold and mildew. It has been clear for over 2000 years that mycotoxins pose a significant threat to human health. If you have a complicated illness that never seems to get better and is worse in a damp environment, you likely have mycotoxin exposure impacting your health. While the symptoms of mycotoxin exposure can be mild or severe, the potential for long-term health problems underscores the importance of prevention and proactive measures to protect yourself and your family.

TOXICANTS

Toxicity is the ability of a substance—a toxicant or poison—to harm humans and animals. It is important to note that toxins and toxicants can affect different individuals differently, depending on their age, health, genetics, and exposure level. Additionally, exposure to multiple toxicants can have additive or synergistic effects, making it even more important to limit exposure to toxicants on a day-to-day basis.

Why am I calling them 'toxicants' rather than 'toxins'? Toxins are poisons from natural sources (like mold, snakes, bacteria, spiders, mushrooms, etc.). Toxicants are man-made chemicals that play a significant role in causing chronic diseases and health problems. Exposure to toxicants is much more of a health concern than toxins for most Americans. While the term 'toxins' is better known, I will use the term 'toxicants' for accuracy. It is hard to pinpoint which toxicants are to blame for causing diabetes, obesity, cardiovascular diseases, autoimmunity, infertility, cancer, and nervous system diseases. 86,000 industrial chemicals are registered as toxic with the EPA and only a fraction of them have been tested for impacts on human health. There is also no study looking at how they impact human health together; experts say that they are probably more dangerous in combination, with disease-causing power greater than the sum of the parts. Additionally, studies on high doses of endocrine-disrupting chemicals (EDCs) in animals cannot predict the effects of low doses, which occur in the range of human exposures and have been proven to cause human diseases and disabilities.

Nobody is exposed to only one toxicant at a time in our polluted environment. Most chemicals have never been tested for human safety because the companies that own the government asserted there wouldn't be enough human exposure to be concerned. *Whoops*, that hasn't been the case at all. In 2005, the Environmental Working Group (ewg.org) tested the umbilical cord blood of newborns and found over 250 different industrial chemicals in the blood. This is especially problematic because these chemicals can cross the placenta, a structure created by a mother to protect the baby from the environment. Do you think newborns have more or fewer chemicals in them now? More, many more.

After birth, we are exposed to more toxic chemicals in the environment. We swim in a toxic soup of potential cancer-causing and hormone-disrupting chemicals. Our food, water, and air are seriously toxic. It is also estimated that one out of every five Americans is exposed every day to the top seven cancer-causing chemicals in personal care products. Your shampoo, conditioner, perfume, lotion, makeup, toothpaste, detergent, etc., most likely contain chemicals that cause cancer and hormone imbalances. 'Fragrance' is becoming known as the 'second-hand smoke' of the 21st century.

We have information about the health impacts of many of these chemicals found in newborns and what they do to humans: many cause nerve and brain damage, cancer, and hormone imbalances. Even more alarming is that much lower amounts of these chemicals are now known to cause health problems than we previously thought.

That means the levels we have been told are 'safe' are unsafe. Plus, many of these toxicants 'bio-accumulate' in fat, which means they are stored in your body. This is especially true if you are not actively supporting your detoxification systems with adequate nutrition or if you are dehydrated or constipated. I could write a whole book about the health impacts of chemical toxicants because I have been researching and treating them for almost twenty years and recently wrote a fifty-page research document for one of the medical labs that tests human exposure. But you want to know the basics rather than boring organic chemistry and biochemistry, right?

THE HARM CAUSED BY MOST TOXICANTS WILL FALL INTO THE FOLLOWING CATEGORIES

Endocrine Disruptors harm the hormone system and knock it out of balance. They often mimic estrogen, decrease testosterone, impair the thyroid gland's function, and interfere with hormone receptors, so you don't recognize or use your hormones properly. A wide range of natural and man-made substances cause endocrine disruption. These substances include pharmaceuticals, dioxin, dioxin-like compounds, polychlorinated biphenyls (PCBs), DDT (and other pesticides), PFAs, and plasticizers like BPA and BPS. BPS is similar to BPA, and companies add it to BPA-free products even though it is roughly ten times more harmful than BPA. Endocrine disruptors are found in almost everything, including everyday products such as plastic bottles, metal food can linings, detergents, fabrics treated with stain and flame retardants, food, toys, cosmetics, personal care products, and pesticides.

Long-term exposure to endocrine disruptors paves the way for lowered fertility, increased endometriosis, and some cancers. Over the past 50 years, there has been a significant decline in sperm count among men worldwide. Studies have found that the average sperm count has decreased by 50–60% over the past five decades. This trend has raised concerns about the potential impact of environmental factors, such as exposure to chemicals and pollutants, on male fertility. My colleague, Dr. Brendan McCarthy, refers to it as 'spermageddon.'

One of the most comprehensive studies on this topic was published in 2017, which analyzed data from over 43,000 men from 50 different countries. The study found that the average sperm count per milliliter of semen decreased from 99 million in 1973 to 47 million in 2011. This decline in sperm count has been linked to various environmental and lifestyle factors, including exposure to endocrine-disrupting chemicals, poor nutrition, sedentary lifestyles, and increased stress levels. In addition to the decline in sperm count, there has also been an increase in the prevalence of other male fertility problems, such as low sperm motility, poor sperm morphology (shape), and decreased sperm volume.

Research conducted by the NIH shows that the most significant risk from exposure to toxicants is during prenatal and infant development when organ and neural systems are forming. But as stated earlier, you encounter these chemicals your whole life and then store them in your bodies in your fat stores, making dysfunction and disease creation much more likely.

Carcinogens are chemicals capable of causing cancer by damaging DNA. Cancer is quickly passing cardiovascular disease to become the number one killer of Americans.

Neurotoxicants are chemicals capable of killing neurons and causing brain damage or impaired brain function. Global dementia cases are forecasted to triple by the year 2050.

Mitochondrial toxicants damage your power centers. Your mitochondria are responsible for producing the energy for your body. If you can't effectively use the food you eat for energy, you cannot build, protect, or repair your body. Additionally, many individuals are affected by associated diseases (i.e., not caused directly or entirely by mitochondrial dysfunction), common aging diseases such as Parkinson's disease, Alzheimer's disease, and many forms of cancer.

Obesogens are chemicals in the environment stimulate your body to become obese. It is estimated that half the US population will be obese by 2030.

HOW ARE YOU EXPOSED?

Your food, air, water, textiles, home goods, and personal care products expose you to these chemical toxicants. Often, one specific chemical will be an obesogen, a hormone disruptor, a carcinogen, and a neurotoxin all at the same time. I won't overwhelm you with all the science stuff, and you should know that National Water Testing recently found more than 300 chemicals in tap water. Many industrial chemicals and additives have never been tested for human safety and hide within "proprietary formulas".

WHY YOU SHOULD ALWAYS CHOOSE ORGANIC

Almost 900 pesticides have been approved in the U.S., including herbicides and insecticides. They can cause neurological problems, including autism spectrum disorder, depression, impulsivity, suicide, anxiety, behavioral problems, poorer short-term memory, impaired motor skills, developmental delays, cardiotoxicity, hormone disruption, diabetes, and cancer. Metabolic syndrome is also worsened by pesticide exposure because it complicates glucose metabolism and increases blood pressure.

WHY MONSANTO HAD TO CHANGE ITS NAME

Glyphosate is one of the main active ingredients in Roundup™, the number-one herbicide in the world. It was created by Monsanto and sprayed on GMO corn, which we feed our livestock and make high fructose corn syrup from, as well as GMO soy and rice. It is also sprayed on conventional wheat fields to increase crop yields and dry the wheat faster with less fungus growth. It has been associated with many chronic diseases.

The World Health Organization classifies glyphosate it as a probable human carcinogen. It also kills off healthy gut flora and increases the risk of Salmonella and C. diff infections. Exposure to glyphosate is associated with autism, autoimmunity, congenital disabilities, and various reproductive issues.

Contaminated ingredients derived from corn, wheat, soy, and rice are found in almost every packaged food in the U.S.

VOLATILE ORGANIC COMPOUNDS (VOCS)

Perhaps the most researched VOC, BTEX is a well-studied combination of Benzene, Toluene, Ethylbenzene, and Xylene air pollution. It is associated with cancer, respiratory issues like asthma, cardiovascular disease, and nervous system issues. Benzene is among the top 20 chemicals most often used in the U.S. and comes from burning coal and oil, motor vehicle exhaust, cigarette smoke, and evaporation from gas stations. People are exposed through inhalation, eating food, and drinking water contaminated with it. In a large U.S. study cited by the CDC, 95% of participants had detectable levels of benzene in their blood.

VOCs are a massive group of chemicals that are toxic to mitochondria and have irrefutable links to cancer, autoimmunity, and other chronic diseases. They are found in outdoor air, as well as indoor air contaminated with artificial fragrances used in clothes detergent, air fresheners, perfumes, skin-care products, hair sprays, cosmetics, lotions, adhesives, aftershave, household cleaners, floor wax, latex, and cleaning chemicals.

FUCK PLASTIC

Phthalates, including DEHP and DEP, are found in lubricants, adhesives, and plasticizers (chemicals used to make plastic more flexible and less breakable). These chemicals are why you never eat food from microwaved plastic containers and only drink warm water out of plastic water bottles if you are dying in the desert. They are also found in car interiors, shower curtains, deodorants, cosmetics, the linings of canned foods, medical devices, the thermal paper used in cash register receipts, and paper money.

Phthalates are well-known endocrine disruptors associated with hormonal imbalances, reproductive problems including early puberty, altered reproductive development, endometriosis, sex anomalies, infertility, congenital disabilities, and breast and skin cancers. They are obesogens and cause obesity and metabolic syndrome issues, including impaired glucose metabolism leading to pre-diabetes and Type II diabetes and increased blood pressure.

Many plasticizers are also neurological toxins linked to low I.Q., neurodevelopmental issues, behavior issues, autism spectrum disorders, and ADHD. Phthalates are toxic to most body systems, including the heart, liver, kidneys, and immune system, and can worsen allergies and asthma.

Microplastic particle pollution is everywhere in the environment; it is estimated that the average person eats five grams of microplastic a week, about the size of a credit card. These particles are bioavailable for uptake into the human bloodstream and are small enough to get inside your cells. Studies on humans and animals recognize that microplastics are cytotoxic, cause oxidative stress inflammatory responses, damage DNA, harm embryos, damage the liver, nerves, and kidneys, and can cause cancer. Microplastics can bioaccumulate in the liver, spleen, kidney, brain, lung, and gut, and the toxicity can be passed onto offspring.

WHY I NEVER EAT ATLANTIC SALMON

Polychlorinated Biphenyls (PCBs) are a class of industrial chemicals widely used as coolants, electrical and heat transfer insulators, plasticizers, waterproofing materials, pigments, and dyes. Production was outlawed in the U.S. in the 1970s, but since they are persistent organic pollutants (POPs), they are still widely found in the environment.

Additionally, the EPA didn't ban ALL production or importation; their website lists 'inadvertent PCBs' as allowed as pigments and dyes, G.E. silicones, vinyl chloride production, and 'unique and unknown' processes. PCBs contaminate water, and fish are a significant exposure in our food chain.

In 2004, Science published the *Global Assessment of Organic Contaminants in Farmed Salmon* and found almost eight times the levels of PCBs in farmed Atlantic salmon than in wild Alaskan salmon. In 2020, an update on foods listed higher amounts of PCBs in wild Atlantic salmon from Norway than in farmed Atlantic salmon. So, I would suggest avoiding eating Atlantic salmon, ever.

PCBs cause cancer, low birth weight, developmental delays, low I.Q., impaired memory, and behavioral and neurological problems, including depression. Endocrine effects include mimicking estrogen, changing sex ratios in children, altering the metabolism of sex steroids in the body, and reducing sperm counts. They upset the balance of thyroid hormones in children and adolescents and disturb the immune system, creating greater disease susceptibility.

THE DEVIL YOU KNOW - BPA

Bisphenols (BPA, BPS, etc.) are produced in large quantities worldwide for PVC and plastics that come in contact with food, including packaging, kitchenware, and the inner coatings of cans and jars. They are easily absorbed by humans orally and through the lungs and skin. The constant daily exposures come predominantly from food packaging, dust, dental materials, thermal paper, toys, and healthcare equipment. Do not hand your children receipts to hold; they are absorbing this through their skin.

Bisphenols are endocrine disruptors, interact with estrogen receptors, and play a role in infertility, early puberty, breast and prostate cancer, and PCOS. They can also cause aggressive behavior, attention deficit, hyperactivity disorder, depression and anxiety, issues with glucose metabolism, obesity, increased blood pressure, hormonal imbalances with endocrine effects on thyroid hormones, and reproductive problems.

BUT WAIT, THERE'S MORE!

Perchlorates are used as food additives and are

found in chlorinated drinking water, milk, and food. They are theoretically thyroid endocrine disruptors and can cause hypothyroidism and negatively affect the growth and cognitive development of fetuses, infants, and young children.

Dioxins are byproducts of bleaching paper, pesticide processing, and when plastics are burned. They are found worldwide in the soil, accumulate in the food chain in fatty tissue, and 90% of human exposure is through eating fish, shellfish, meat, and dairy products. Another exposure is through infant diapers, tampons, and other sanitary products. Dioxins are highly toxic and known to cause cancer, miscarriage, congenital disabilities, endocrine issues, reproductive problems, immune system dysregulation, neurological damage, and developmental delays.

Tetrachloroethylene (PCE) and Perchloroethylene (PERC) are the most common chemicals used in dry cleaning. They are known carcinogens, reproductive toxicants, and neurotoxins associated with adverse effects on cognition, mood and behavioral problems, sleep, and an increased risk of drug use.

Perfluorinated compounds (PFCs), including Per- and Polyfluoroalkyl substances (PFAs), are pervasive environmental toxicants with extreme persistence and bioaccumulative potential. That means they are everywhere, and they are a real bitch to get out of your body, so avoiding them is key. PFAs, referred to as 'forever chemicals,' do not break down in the environment, and the only way to get them out is to bleed them out. That is how stubborn they are. They are found in textiles, food packaging, drinking water, and non-stick cookware.

Health impacts include impaired fertility and fetal

development, pre-diabetes, high cholesterol, impaired lipid metabolism, damage to the endocrine system, toxicity to the liver and immune system, and they cause cancer and ADHD.

Polycyclic Aromatic Hydrocarbons (PAHs) from burning fossil fuels and other organic matter are associated with lung cancer, asthma, allergies, and metabolic syndrome components, including increased blood pressure, glucose and lipid metabolism issues, and obesity. These are the guys likely responsible for air pollution increasing the risk of diabetes.

Wow! If you aren't consciously avoiding them, you are likely exposed to most of these chemicals daily. They are very likely making you and your family sick. That is why I am so passionate about this topic and created The Wilde Vitality Detoxification Program. It is designed to mobilize and excrete most of the toxicants listed above from where they are stored in fat and other body tissues. When you implement the processes in this book and change your behaviors, you will decrease your exposure to these chemicals. The most critical element of environmental medicine is to not get poisoned in the first place.

HEAVY METALS AND OTHER TOXIC METALS

Heavy and toxic metals like mercury, lead, cadmium, and arsenic are a more complicated story because removing them requires a more in-depth process called chelation, which must be done under the care of an experienced professional.

These pollutants are true villains. They cause nerve damage and DNA damage, increasing the risk of dementia and cancer. Heavy metals clog up receptors and keep the body from normal functioning. They are toxic to all systems of the body.

Some individuals are more sensitive to heavy metal exposure compared to others. The more toxicants accumulate in our bodies, the greater the chance of experiencing related illnesses determined by our genes and heritage. Most conventional testing only tests for acute metal exposure, or what you are exposed to on an average day. A challenged urine test is necessary to get the best idea of your "body burden." Environmental medicine doctors refer to the amount of heavy metals and other toxicants you have stored in your body as your "body burden." Determining the body's exact level of heavy metals is impossible because many are stored and bound up in tissues like bones, fat, and the sheaths around nerves. The best testing available is a *Challenged and Timed Urine Collection*, which requires a pharmaceutical chelating agent (a drug that pulls heavy metals out of tissues) to be taken orally or by IV. All urine produced is collected for a set time, usually 6–24 hours. This test depends on the body's ability to excrete metals effectively through the kidneys, and considering many people with heavy metal toxicity may also have compromised detoxification abilities, this poses an issue in the exact determination of levels in the body. The chelating agents also have different affinities for different metals.

Do the exact levels matter? No. Not really, because we all have heavy metals and toxins in our bodies. Is it always necessary to remove them? Not necessarily. The FDA has approved chelation therapy for coronary artery disease, and it can be very beneficial in severe chronic diseases like autoimmunity and cancer when other therapies have been used and haven't produced the desired results. In my clinical experience, when you chelate people correctly, they feel better.

Chelation therapy is the ultimate detoxification for the body to get rid of metals. Prescription chelating drugs like EDTA and/or DMSA are administered to bind to metals in the blood and tissues. The chelating substance can be administered intravenously (IV) or as a pill. Once the drug attaches to the metal, the body can eliminate it through the excretion processes in the liver and kidneys. Due to the expertise needed to chelate metals out of the body, you want to find an expert who will not only remove the heavy metals safely and effectively but will also support your body and protect it from the damage that can be caused when the metals start to move.

I recommend this therapy to my clients, but it usually isn't a first-line therapy. Chelation needs to be done with a licensed, trained professional, and you want to be sure your practitioner is giving you nutritional, liver, kidney, and mineral support in addition to glutathione when it is being performed.

Otherwise, find a different practitioner. The same applies to dentists removing mercury fillings. If all they do is give you oxygen, find another provider who understands the complexity of the process and prescribes DMSA during and after the procedures. Chelating agents will protect you from exposure to mercury during the process by automatically binding to the aerosolized mercury and chelating it out of the body so you do not store it in your tissues.

If you want to give your future children the healthiest and best life possible, detoxification and chelation therapy should be done 2-3 years before you plan to conceive.

WARNING: Do not chelate when there is a

possibility that you can become pregnant, are pregnant, or are breastfeeding.

Toxic and Heavy Metals can be found everywhere in the environment. Common exposures include:

• **Lead** – The Proceedings of the National Academy of Sciences estimate that over 170 million Americans alive today were exposed to five-plus times the current safe reference level of lead, resulting in 824,097,690 lost I.Q. points, or 2.6 per person as of 2015. In some cities, lead is everywhere in the environment, largely due to leaded gas, paint, car batteries, lead-based ceramic glazes, ammunition, water pipes, and drinking water. It is also found in foods and cosmetics, including long-lasting lipstick and hair dyes. Mushrooms have a high ability to accumulate toxic elements, including lead and other heavy metals. Lead gets stored in your bones, liver, kidneys, and brain and can cause neurological problems, developmental delays, anemia, hypertension, and cardiovascular disease.

• **Mercury-** Mercury exposures occur mainly through consuming fish and shellfish, high fructose corn syrup (HFCS), mushrooms, and dental amalgams (silver fillings). They can cause neurological problems, including anxiety, mood swings, memory issues, tremors, depression, numbness and tingling, loss of motor skills, vision and speech impairment, muscle weakness, trouble walking, developmental delays, and kidney damage, along with metabolic syndrome associations with obesity, blood pressure, and glucose metabolism problems.

• **Arsenic** - Arsenic exposure from drinking water sources worldwide is associated with an increased risk of developing chronic diseases, including metabolic diseases. Food sources of arsenic include seafood, rice, rice products, mushrooms, and poultry (non-organic). It can cause cancer, liver damage, rash, insulin resistance, obesity, inflammation, Type II diabetes, peripheral neuropathy, night blindness, and cardiovascular disease, including high blood pressure, endothelial dysfunction, and elevated cholesterol.

• **Cadmium** - Cadmium exposure from industrial and agricultural sources can be inhaled or ingested. Foods high in cadmium include shellfish, kidneys, liver, mushrooms, grains, and rood crops. It can cause prostate, breast, lung, pancreatic, and kidney cancers, lung, liver, and kidney damage, osteoporosis, and anemia. It is a mitochondrial toxin associated with blood pressure, glucose, and lipid metabolism issues.

• **Aluminum** - Aluminum exposure often occurs from processed foods, sunscreens, toothpaste, antiperspirants, and pharmaceuticals such as antacids and buffered aspirin, as well as drinking water, vaccines, aluminum cans, aluminum foil, aluminum cookware, and baking powder (so buy Al-free). Aluminum is a recognized neurotoxin that affects over 200 important biological reactions and causes negative effects on brain development, neurotransmitter production and reception, gene expression, and inflammation. It is associated with Alzheimer's disease, Parkinson's disease, multiple sclerosis, breast cancer, reproductive toxicity, impaired kidney function, and learning and memory impairments.

• **Other metals** - Other toxic metals include antimony, barium, beryllium, bismuth, cesium, gadolinium, nickel, palladium, platinum, tellurium, thallium, thorium, tin, tungsten, and uranium.

Remember Flint, Michigan? Heavy metal toxicity results in alopecia (hair loss), osteoporosis, cardiovascular disease, depression, dermatitis, poor wound healing, fatigue, gastrointestinal issues, hypertension, immune problems, impaired glucose tolerance, inflammation, cognitive impairment, poor memory, anemia, renal dysfunction, cardiovascular disease and hypertension, autoimmune disorders, nervous system issues, kidney issues, and the list goes on.

Heavy metals will stress your system, making it weaker and more likely to experience many diseases. One way to decrease exposure is to stop eating tuna and other large game fish. I know; there goes sushi date night. Do you want to give up spicy tuna and decrease your dementia risk? Or not? Identify your priorities and choose your health adventure.

RADIATION AND EMF

Everyone knows that radiation causes cancer. This fact is undisputed, but we aren't fully aware of other invisible wave frequencies' effects on health. In today's world, electromagnetic fields (EMFs) are everywhere. EMFs are constantly in our lives, from television and radio signals to Wi-Fi networks and cell phones. As we continue to rely more and more on technology, concerns have arisen about the potential health impacts of exposure to EMFs and cell phone radiation.

EMFs are a type of energy that is generated by the movement of electrically charged particles. These fields can be natural, such as the Earth's magnetic field, or man-made, such as those generated by power lines and electronic devices. Cell phone radiation is a specific EMF emitted by cell phones and other wireless devices. This radiation is also known as radiofrequency radiation or microwave radiation and can heat the tissue, kind of like mini microwaves. Have you ever noticed that your head starts to hurt or your ear gets hot when you hold your phone against your head?

There is an ongoing debate about the health impacts of EMFs and cell phone radiation. While some studies have suggested that exposure to these fields can lead to various health problems, others have found no evidence of harm. However, reading the documentation on your cell phone will instruct you to hold the phone at least 3 inches away from your body when it is in use.

One of the most significant concerns about exposure to EMFs and cell phone radiation is the potential for cancer. The World Health Organization's International Agency for Research on Cancer (IARC) has classified EMFs as "possibly carcinogenic to humans." This classification was based on evidence from studies that showed an increased risk of brain tumors in people who used cell phones for more than 30 minutes per day over ten years or more.

Other studies, however, have found no link between EMFs and cancer. For example, a National Institutes of Health study found no association between cell phone use and brain cancer. However, the researchers did note that there was some evidence of a potential link between cell phone use and a rare type of tumor called acoustic neuroma, a tumor of the auditory nerve. This cranial nerve grows right out of the brain.

There is also convincing evidence to suggest that

exposure to EMFs and cell phone radiation could negatively impact reproductive health. A study published in the journal *Fertility and Sterility* found that men who used laptops with Wi-Fi for more than four hours per day had significantly lower sperm counts and motility than men who did not use laptops with Wi-Fi.

Another study published in the Journal of Reproductive Medicine found that men who used cell phones for more than four hours per day had significantly lower sperm counts and motility than men who used cell phones for less than two hours per day. Your cell phone is almost always on, and carrying it in your pocket (next to your testicles, if you have them) or in your bra (if you wear one) is no bueno. Another study showed that smartphone use significantly increased breast cancer risk, especially if the phone was close to the breasts. So, please don't carry your smartphone on your body; put it in your purse, backpack, bike messenger bag, fanny pack, or Indiana Jones satchel.

There is also some concern about the potential neurological effects of exposure to EMFs and cell phone radiation. Studies have found that exposure to these fields can lead to changes in brain function, including changes in memory, attention, and reaction times. Some researchers have suggested that these changes could be linked to an increased risk of conditions such as Alzheimer's and Parkinson's disease. Another potential health impact of exposure to EMFs and cell phone radiation is sleep disturbances which we know cause all kinds of problems with the body.

Studies have found that exposure to these fields can lead to changes in sleep patterns, including decreased sleep quality and increased nighttime awakenings. This could be because EMFs and cell phone radiation can interfere with the production of melatonin, a hormone that helps regulate sleep.

Of course, there is rational concern about the potential health impacts of EMFs and cell phone radiation on children. Screens are addictive and create mental and emotional issues that throw in EMF and radiation, which is even more cause for concern. Children are more vulnerable to the effects of these fields because their brains and bodies are still developing. Some studies have suggested that exposure to these fields increases the risk of behavioral problems, developmental delays, and other health problems in children, let alone future hormonal and reproductive issues, from tablets on their laps.

Given the potential health impacts of EMFs and cell phone radiation, it's natural to want to protect yourself from these fields without being a complete Luddite and getting a flip phone. One simple step is to reduce your use of cell phones and other wireless devices. We will talk more about this in the Digital Detox section.

When you do use these devices, try to keep them away from your body. For example, you can use a headset or speakerphone instead of holding your phone to your ear. You can also use airplane mode or turn off your phone when you're not using it to reduce your exposure. Next, limit your exposure to other EMF sources, such as Wi-Fi networks, power lines, and electronic devices. You can do this by turning off your Wi-Fi at night when you're not using it, avoiding using your laptop on your lap, and keeping your electronic devices at a distance when you're not using them. There are a lot of products out there, like grounding pads, Q-links, etc., that are touted as protection against EMF radiation. I don't make any specific recommendations. I urge you to do your own research into how important it is to block your smart meter and decrease Bluetooth use.

Dr. Bill Rea, MD, a pioneering cardiovascular surgeon who more or less invented environmental medicine, founded the Environmental Health Center, Dallas, and made green building mainstream. I did a medical rotation with him and was surprised when he saw some patients with the lights off because he recognized EMFs were negatively impacting their health. If that brilliant man gave EMF toxicity credence, then I was going to, too. Like any toxic exposure, avoidance is key and helps decrease your overall burden.

If you have been struggling with your health and interventions that should help you feel better haven't been having the impact you hoped for, toxins are likely making everything more difficult. In that case, take a deeper look at all kinds of toxic exposures from molds, radiation, emf, and non-metallic and metallic toxicity because something is standing in the way of your body's inherent ability to heal. The best thing about detoxing is you feel so much better.

I know. That was a lot. Stress, inflammation, and toxicity are three interrelated factors that are part of a vicious cycle of dysfunction driving chronic disease development.

Stress, be it physical, chemical (toxic), or psychological, has been linked to the development of chronic inflammation.

Inflammation is stressful and toxic in its own right.

Toxic exposures to the 86,000 industrial toxicants build up in your body and interfere with the normal functioning of cells and tissues, leading to oxidative stress and inflammation, cell damage, and the development of chronic diseases such as cancer, diabetes, heart disease, infertility, and dementia. I hope that understanding some of the science behind toxicity will inspire you to regularly detoxify and change your habits meaningfully, not only for yourself but for everyone you love.

REFERENCES

This isn't a scientific paper, it is for people without medical, scientific, or technical backgrounds, and I will therefore not adhere to proper citation protocol because it can be confusing and difficult to access. For those of you who wish to look more into scientific papers, here are the PubMed National Institutes of Health and National Library of Medicine Reference Links:

https://www.ncbi.nlm.nih.gov/pmc/articles/PMC7044178/

https://pubmed.ncbi.nlm.nih.gov/24945191/

https://pubmed.ncbi.nlm.nih.gov/25813067/

https://www.ncbi.nlm.nih.gov/pmc/articles/PMC7664834/

https://www.ncbi.nlm.nih.gov/pmc/articles/PMC8701112/

https://www.ncbi.nlm.nih.gov/pmc/articles/PMC7460375/

https://www.ncbi.nlm.nih.gov/pmc/articles/PMC3371394/

https://pubmed.ncbi.nlm.nih.gov/32178293/

https://www.ncbi.nlm.nih.gov/pmc/articles/PMC1226284/

https://www.ncbi.nlm.nih.gov/pmc/articles/PMC9145289/

https://pubmed.ncbi.nlm.nih.gov/17002710/

https://pubmed.ncbi.nlm.nih.gov/30894343/

https://pubmed.ncbi.nlm.nih.gov/34231153/

https://www.ncbi.nlm.nih.gov/pmc/articles/PMC1519588/

https://www.ncbi.nlm.nih.gov/pmc/articles/PMC5635510/

https://pubmed.ncbi.nlm.nih.gov/26121921/

https://www.ncbi.nlm.nih.gov/pmc/articles/PMC8878656/

https://www.ncbi.nlm.nih.gov/pmc/articles/PMC6712572/

https://pubmed.ncbi.nlm.nih.gov/35367073/

https://pubmed.ncbi.nlm.nih.gov/25635985/

https://www.ncbi.nlm.nih.gov/pmc/articles/PMC3268745/

https://www.ncbi.nlm.nih.gov/pmc/articles/PMC9603407/

https://www.ncbi.nlm.nih.gov/pmc/articles/PMC3693132/

https://www.ncbi.nlm.nih.gov/pmc/articles/PMC4958597/

https://www.ncbi.nlm.nih.gov/pmc/articles/PMC9150370/

https://www.ncbi.nlm.nih.gov/pmc/articles/PMC8727895/

PART III
THE WILDE WAY TO DETOX

CHAPTER 11
HOW TO DETOX

If the previous section outraged you, scared you or stressed you out, do not despair! I developed The Wilde Vitality Detoxification Program to help address toxicity in the most effective way you can without a prescription. While exposure to a tremendous amount of toxicity is causing increased rates of chronic disease, the human body is an incredibly resilient miracle. If you give it what it needs, it will work even better to detoxify the chemical toxicants you are exposed to. In reality, you can't go live in a bubble and avoid all the toxicants and pollutants in the environment. Even if you did, the bubble would most likely be made from plastic!

The previous chapter most likely convinced you of the need to detoxify your body when you realized how many harmful chemicals you are exposed to daily. Detox was originally most well known as a treatment for drug addicts or alcoholics. That is no longer the case, as many people have encountered the idea of 'detoxing' to remove chemicals from their body to support their health.

If you eat non-organic food, drink bottled or tap water, regularly eat at restaurants, use conventional cosmetics, household cleaners, and personal care products, and breathe unfiltered city air, I know your body is stressed by toxicants.

HOW DOES DETOXIFICATION WORK?

Detoxing, or detoxification, is a process that helps to eliminate poisonous and waste substances from the body. The process aids in maintaining optimal health because the body cannot function well if it is full of poisons running around doing damage. Over time, toxicity will speed your progress toward aging and disease. The detoxification phases are complex and use several organ systems, including the skin, liver, kidneys, lungs, and digestive systems, to remove toxicity from the body.

DETOXIFICATION PHASES I, II, AND III

Blood filtration is one of the most essential functions performed by the liver. As the blood is filtered, the harmful parts are detoxified through Phases I, II, and III of the detoxification process.

Phase I, II, and III detoxification in the liver and kidneys is a multi-step process of breaking down and eliminating harmful substances from the body. Phase I is the first step in liver detoxification and involves the oxidation, reduction, and hydroxylation of harmful substances to make them more water-soluble and easier to eliminate.

This is done by a group of enzymes called the cytochrome P450 system. Phase I can neutralize unwanted chemical compounds, but more often it produces intermediate forms that are more toxic than the original compound and need to be altered by phase II as quickly as possible.

Every metabolic pathway in your body is supported by vitamins and minerals acting as co-factors. When you are depleted in co-factors with time, age, and toxicity, your body's processes slow down. The cytochrome P450 system requires several co-factors to function properly.

Some of the key nutrients involved in this process include:

- **Magnesium:** Essential for activating cytochrome P450 enzymes and their ability to metabolize harmful substances.

- **Vitamin B6:** Helps to regulate the activity of the cytochrome P450 system and supports its function.

- **Vitamin C:** A powerful antioxidant that can recycle other antioxidants, helps protect the liver, and supports the cytochrome P450 system.

- **Zinc:** Involved in regulating the cytochrome P450 system and is necessary for the proper functioning of these enzymes.

The need for cofactors is the main reason why I don't recommend fasting for detoxification. You need nutrients for your detox systems to work. In phase II, the modified substances from phase I are conjugated, or combined, with other substances such as glucuronic acid, sulfur, or amino acids, making them even more water-soluble and easier to excrete from the body. Nutrients to support Phase II include:

- **Glutathione:** It is the number one antioxidant produced by your body, helps to protect the liver cells, and supports phase II liver detoxification. It is also amazing for everything from cancer to hangovers.

- **N-Acetyl Cysteine (NAC):** It is a precursor to glutathione as it helps support phase II liver detoxification by increasing glutathione levels. The FDA has outlawed it, and it will soon no longer be included in over-the-counter supplements.

- **Vitamin B2:** Riboflavin is necessary to convert harmful substances into water-soluble compounds that can be eliminated from the body. It is also involved in your energy production and methylation pathways, making your pee fluorescent yellow.

• **Vitamin B3, (Niacin):** Niacin produces energy in the liver and is necessary for the proper functioning of phase II liver detoxification. If you have heard of the NAD+ supplement, it is just an expensive form of Niacin.

• **Folate:** It supports glutathione production and is necessary for the proper functioning of phase II liver detoxification and methylation. People with an epigenetic MTHFR (methylenetetrahydrofolate reductase) defect cannot properly activate their folate.

• **Vitamin B12:** It is involved in the production of energy in the liver and is necessary for the proper functioning of phase II liver detoxification.

• **Magnesium:** It is essential again to activate the enzymes involved in phase II liver detoxification. Magnesium is one of the more common nutrient deficiencies among Americans. It is an especially important supplement because it plays a role in almost everything the body does.

In Phase III, the conjugated substances from Phase II are eliminated from the body through bile in stool, urine, and sweat.

GI DETOXIFICATION

Twenty-five percent of detoxification occurs in intestinal lining cells, where chemicals and other dietary toxins and contaminants are rendered harmless and excreted or are reabsorbed and hitch a ride to the liver. Once the liver metabolizes waste products and toxicants, they are released into the intestines through bile and the gallbladder. The primary function of the intestines is to absorb molecules, and therefore, potential toxicants can be reabsorbed into the bloodstream if you are not eliminating (pooping) regularly.

Constipation is a severe issue for many reasons, but the reabsorption of toxins is one of the most concerning. You should have at least one well-formed and easy-to-pass bowel movement a day. A diet high in fibrous, non-starchy vegetables and non-processed foods is a good start toward bowel health. You will probably have the best bowel movements of your life when you experience the detox I designed.

Your large intestine has a critical role in your body's water balance. If you aren't drinking enough, your intestines will absorb water, causing hard, dry, difficult-to-pass stools. That is why drinking enough water to help flush your tissues and kidneys, replenish sweat, and get enough fiber so you are pooping at least once daily is necessary during the detox. Otherwise, you can reabsorb the toxins back into the body after your liver worked so hard to get them out!

One way to reduce the effects of toxicants and mycotoxins is to support digestive health. This can be achieved by consuming fiber-rich foods, prebiotics, and probiotics. Fiber helps promote the growth of beneficial bacteria in the gut, which can help break down and eliminate mycotoxins. Prebiotics are substances that nourish the beneficial bacteria in the gut, while probiotics are live microorganisms that can help restore the gut bacteria's balance. Consuming foods rich in prebiotics, such as garlic, onions, leeks, asparagus, and bananas, can help support digestive health and reduce the effects of mycotoxins.

Several binders have been studied for their effectiveness in binding mycotoxins in the gut and reducing their absorption into the bloodstream. Some of the most commonly recommended binders for mycotoxins and toxicants include:

• **Activated charcoal:** It is a highly porous material that binds toxins in the digestive tract, preventing them from being absorbed into the bloodstream.

• **Bentonite clay:** Bentonite clay is another highly porous material commonly used as a binder for mycotoxins. It has a high negative charge, which allows it to attract and bind positively charged toxins.

• **Glucomannan:** Glucomannan is a soluble fiber in the Konjac plant's root. It has been shown to bind to mycotoxins in the gut and reduce their absorption into the bloodstream.

• **Modified citrus pectin:** Modified citrus pectin is a modified form of pectin that increases its ability to bind to toxins. It has been shown to bind to various mycotoxins in the gut and prevent their absorption.

Don't take binders with other supplements because they are so good at binding; they will decrease your absorption of other nutrients.

It is important to note that while these binders have shown promise in reducing the absorption of mycotoxins in the gut, they should not be relied upon as a sole strategy for dealing with mold exposure. It is critical to address the underlying source of the mold and take steps to remediate it. In more challenging cases, you may also wish to consult a qualified healthcare practitioner for individualized advice on mycotoxin exposure in the overall scheme of what is happening with your health.

KIDNEY DETOXIFICATION

The kidneys are the unsung heroes of our bodies, working tirelessly to filter out toxins and waste products from our blood. In phase III detoxification, also known as the 'elimination' phase, the kidneys play a crucial role in the excretion of water-soluble toxins processed by the liver.

This involves the transport of these toxins out of the liver and into the bloodstream, where the kidneys filter and ultimately excrete them in the urine. The kidneys also play a role in maintaining the body's acid-base balance, which is important for proper detoxification. Drinking enough water is even more important than usual when detoxifying because it helps reduce the stress on the kidneys.

Kidney damage leads to various health issues, including chronic kidney disease and renal failure. When the kidneys are compromised, the consequences can be devastating because wastes build up in the blood and the fluid dynamics of the body are compromised, resulting in swelling and other uncomfortable symptoms, including nausea, vomiting, loss of appetite, fatigue, weakness, sleep problems, brain fog, and muscle cramps.

The insidious effects of mycotoxins, cadmium, and other toxicants on kidney function are well documented in scientific research, and you can take proactive steps to mitigate their harmful effects by minimizing your exposure. By decreasing how many toxins and toxicants you are exposed to, you decrease the stress on your liver and kidneys. The first step in protecting your kidneys is ensuring that you are properly hydrated. The second step is to identify and eliminate the source of toxic exposures.

This may involve removing mold from your living space or reducing exposure to other environmental toxicants. Filter your air and water, and support your overall health with a balanced diet and regular exercise. Are you starting to recognize a pattern? Food, water, and movement? But why stop there? There are several natural supplements and herbs that have been shown to help protect kidney function from toxicants. With its anti-inflammatory properties, turmeric can help reduce inflammation in the kidneys and protect against damage. Milk thistle, another herb with powerful protective properties, has been shown to help reduce the risk of liver and renal damage from toxicants.

SKIN DETOXIFICATION

Our skin's role in detoxification is critical and yet commonly overlooked. If you have any skin issues, especially acne, your skin needs more support to perform its detoxification process better, namely, sweating.

If you don't sweat, that is a big, red warning light with sirens. The skin is the body's largest organ and plays a significant contribution in removing all sorts of toxicants from your system. Some of the sickest people I have seen in practice are those who don't sweat.

Your skin can easily sweat out several liters of fluid when functioning correctly. That fluid, sweat, will carry toxicants out of the body. The best ways to sweat are through exercise, detoxifying baths (like Epsom salt baths), or using a dry sauna. I do not recommend using a steam sauna because most do not use purified water. When you take a steam sauna or hot shower, the toxicants and pollutants in the water become airborne and can be breathed in and absorbed into the body. If you are trying to detoxify, the last thing you want to do is add more toxicants to your system. When you do sweat, be sure to shower as soon as possible so you don't reabsorb the toxins you just got rid of. If you want to take your detox game to the next level, purify the water you bathe in by installing a shower filter.

A DIFFERENT KIND OF BUCKET LIST

Your body normally has at least one overwhelmed detox step or system, which leads to the buildup of those terrible toxicants and contributes to the health problems we already discussed. When your body encounters more chemicals than it can detoxify and get rid of, it has to store them somewhere.

Often, the best the body can do is store toxicants in fat deposits. Fat is the best option to insulate the body from the oxidative and poisonous effects of chemicals, and many toxins are lipophilic anyway. Think of your body as a bucket with a spigot closed at the bottom. Whenever you eat non-organic food, drink from a plastic bottle, use chemical air fresheners or room sprays, light a candle from that place in the mall, and use fabric softener and dryer sheets, you add chemicals to your bucket. You are adding to your overall "body burden."

To continue the metaphor, when your bucket is full and starts to overflow, that is when you get physical symptoms of disease. Everyone is sensitive to these chemicals. They are carcinogens, endocrine disruptors, and neurotoxins.

Some of my clients don't even notice chemical smells. The difference between people who notice chemically caused symptoms and those who don't is a bit complicated, but it is based upon how big their bucket is and how often they open the spigot on the bottom to let the poisons out.

Detoxification opens the spigot, or the emunctories. The emunctories are your Phases of detox, and the organs or structures of the body that are responsible for eliminating waste products and other toxicants.

Let's be real; if you live on this planet, you will benefit from a detox program and from decreasing the chemical stress on your body.

CHAPTER 12: HOW TO CHOOSE THE BEST WAY TO DETOX

In my professional opinion, detoxification is essential. You can see millions of social media posts urging you to detox with different cleanses at the turn of the year, so how do you choose which one is best for you? This chapter was written to educate you about how to choose an effective detox that is worth your time, energy, and money.

JUICE CLEANSES AND THE MASTER CLEANSE

Juice cleanses or liquid-only diets are common fads for detoxification. The idea behind juice cleanses is to flush out toxins from the body while giving the digestive system a rest from heavy foods like meats and starches. Some juice cleanse plans involve drinking only liquid throughout the duration. Others may include light food intake as a snack or meal. Some last for a few days, while others can last for weeks.

The Master Cleanse, for example, instructs people to limit their daily food and water intake to 6 to 12 glasses of water mixed with lemon juice, cayenne pepper, and maple syrup. The "diet" lasts ten or more days and is a "wet fast" because no food is eaten.

Juice cleanses and the Master Cleanse are a good rest for the digestive system and may help normalize gut function. I am not, however, a fan of either cleanse. They can mobilize toxins due to not eating and fat being burned for energy, a process called lipolysis.

When fat is burned, any stored toxicants are released from fat stores. This is a desirable outcome, and I recommend it in my own detoxification program, but when you are fasting, the body doesn't have the needed cofactors like glycine, magnesium, and B-6 in high enough stores to support the body in removing the toxicants.

Think of it like a prison riot. Inmates (toxicants) escape from where they are being securely held (fat stores), but they cannot exit the prison because the liver doesn't have the cofactors necessary for phases I and II. The inmates can then create havoc, causing damage and mayhem in the form of DNA and tissue damage from oxidative stress. Since they can't escape, they just get locked up again after causing trouble.

Consuming only fruit and vegetable-based juices for three days isn't harmful to a healthy person, but a prolonged duration can impact health due to deficient protein intake. Additionally, a juice cleanse doesn't contain any fiber, which won't help eliminate toxins by binding them in the gut. Protein and fiber intake are vital to the body's long-term detoxification process.

FASTING

Fasting is a dietary intervention in which an individual restricts calorie intake for a certain period to promote various health benefits. Autophagy is a cellular process in which the body degrades and recycles damaged or unnecessary cellular components, and it is thought to be one of the mechanisms by which fasting might benefit health.

Studies have shown that fasting can increase autophagy and provide health benefits such as improved insulin sensitivity, reduced oxidative stress, and reduced inflammation. However, fasting should not be considered a cure-all, and more research is needed to fully understand its effects on health and the optimal fasting regimen for various health conditions. Additionally, fasting may not be suitable for everyone, especially individuals with certain medical conditions, pregnant or breastfeeding women, and underweight individuals. I am not an expert in fasting, but I have seen amazing health benefits from its proper use. I do not recommend it for long-term detoxification purposes.

IONIC FOOT BATHS

These foot baths claim to pull toxins out of your feet, as illustrated by the water changing color during the therapy. These may work, but studies have been done on the water before and after and found no release of toxicants to cause the water change. In fact, running water through the bath without feet in it will also cause the water color to change. I have colleagues who disagree and say they have research that it helps detox kids with autism. Can the foot baths help detox? Maybe they would function as part of Phase III detox, and you need to upregulate phase I and phase II for it to really work.

FOOT PATCHES OR DETOX STICKERS

Manufacturers of detox-based foot patches, stickers, and pads claim that these products extract or draw out toxins from the body while the wearer sleeps. There aren't any scientific studies that have been published that show whether detox foot pads work or not. Some of the thickest skin on your body is on your feet, so it would be challenging to pull the toxins through all those layers of skin and be effective.

ZEOLITES

Zeolites have been studied for their potential use in detoxification, specifically in removing heavy metals and other toxins from the body. Some studies have shown that zeolites can bind to heavy metals such as lead, mercury, and cadmium and absorb organic toxins such as benzene and toluene.

Research on using zeolites for detoxification has largely focused on animal models and in vitro studies, with limited clinical evidence supporting their effectiveness in humans. One study published in the Journal of Toxicology and Environmental Health found that zeolite supplementation reduced the levels of heavy metals in the blood of rats exposed to lead, suggesting that zeolites may have the potential to be a detoxifying agent.

This is great if you are eating lead paint or still wearing long-lasting red lipstick (yep... there's lead in that). Zeolites aren't going to remove heavy metals from where they are stored; they just keep you from storing any that you are currently exposed to. They have been used in detoxification as binders in the gut and possibly the circulatory system, but they won't do the whole job alone.

THE WILDE VITALITY DETOXIFICATION PROGRAM

The supplementation packets and detoxification powders we provide in the Wilde Vitality Detoxification Program have been specifically designed to open up your 'spigot' and let 'er flow! Buh-bye, toxicants and poisons!

I created the supplementation protocol to give you the necessary amino acids, vitamins, and minerals for your detox phases. These ingredients function largely like hardware for the proper functioning of your organs. They also contain bioflavonoids, polyphenols, herbs, and other substances that work like software and help program your detox system to function optimally.

Detoxification programs can often stir up toxicity, and the resulting symptoms are uncomfortable. I was there when medical detoxification was pioneered, and one of my teachers detoxed people way too hard and fast. Those first patients experienced a lot of negative side effects. No matter how happy they were to get the toxins out, the process sucked. I learned from his mistakes, and my protocol has several redundancies to ensure that all of your detox processes and emunctories are supported, and the likelihood of having unpleasant side effects is minimized.

Plus, you get to eat! I don't restrict how much you eat; I recommend what foods to consume. The supplement protocol is coupled with specific dietary recommendations that lower your inflammation, normalize your blood sugar, support your digestion, and instigate the burning of fat and the mobilization of toxicants from your tissues.

The process includes lifestyle recommendations, habit retraining, and life hacks to support you through the best detoxification you can do at home without a prescription.

CAUTION: NOT EVERYONE SHOULD DETOX

The world is a toxic place, filled with a mind-blowing amount of pollutants and toxicants that are harmful to health. You would think everyone would benefit from a detox if done correctly, but that's not true.

The one group that should not detoxify is pregnant and lactating women. I repeat: you do not want to detoxify while pregnant or lactating! For women of childbearing age, detoxifying before becoming pregnant can help decrease your baby's exposure to toxicants and improve their health if done long enough before conception and with professional help.

I detoxed for a year in preparation before I conceived my son. Mothers build babies out of their own bodies and pass some of their body burden and toxicants on to their children. The less you give your kids, the better, but it must be done long enough before conception otherwise you can cause birth defects.

Young children should only detoxify when there are no other options and under the care of an experienced professional.

People with a history of eating disorders, kidney failure, liver failure, or advanced cancer may benefit from detoxification. Still, they should do it under the care of a medical professional who is well-trained and experienced in detoxification and environmental medicine; otherwise, their health issues are likely to get worse rather than better.

PART IV
HOW TO LIVE YOUR BEST LIFE

CHAPTER 13: YOU ARE WHAT YOU EAT: DON'T BE FAKE, FAST, CHEAP, EASY, OR TOXIC

Thousands of diet books have been published over the years, all claiming to have answers for your health. The worldwide diet industry market size was valued at $175 billion dollars in 2022. With obesity rates growing annually, these interventions don't seem to be effective. In my opinion, the best food choices are those that help you feel vital, healthy, and energetic and it is different for everyone. The Wilde Vitality Detoxification Program helps you get in touch with your body and understand what diet is truly best for your optimal health and wellness. It teaches you to make decisions based on how you feel after you eat, rather than eating to change how you feel.

Let's start with some food basics to set you up for long-term success.

EAT WILDE: DIETARY GUIDELINES – TRUE CLEAN EATING

RULE #1: WHENEVER POSSIBLE, CHOOSE ORGANIC FOR ALL FOODS

I go much more into depth about this in the course I created, but suffice it to say that while organic isn't perfect, it is much less toxic than the alternative.

RULE #2: STRUCTURE YOUR MEALS

Choose wisely when you build your plate of food. Plant-based diets support health and wellness. I am a proponent of eating as many plants as possible. Don't get me wrong. I am against veganism, as the most ill people I see in my office are often vegans.

When building your meals, 60–70% of your plate should be low-glycemic fruits and vegetables. 20–30% should be high-quality protein, and the rest should be high-quality fats.

RULE #3: CHOOSE YOUR CARBOHYDRATES WISELY

The number one component of clean eating is choosing organic fruits, vegetables, nuts, and seeds as carbohydrate sources. Plants are packed with essential vitamins, minerals, antioxidants, fiber, and prebiotics essential for good health.

Organic fruits and vegetables should make up the bulk of your carbohydrate intake. I challenge you to eat ten servings of low-glycemic fruits and vegetables daily and watch your health improve. Will you accept my challenge?

Fruits and vegetables are well known for their nutrient density and health benefits, but several lesser-known benefits make them even more essential to a healthy diet. First, fruits and vegetables are rich in antioxidants, which help protect the body against cellular damage caused by free radicals which are produced by all those toxicants you read about in the last section.

Antioxidants have been shown to reduce the risk of chronic diseases such as cancer, heart disease, and diabetes. In addition, they have anti-inflammatory properties that can help reduce the risk of chronic inflammation, which, as you now know, is one of the main drivers of disease and poor health.

Fruits and non-starchy vegetables are also rich in fiber, which helps promote healthy digestion and regular bowel movements. This can help reduce the risk of constipation, diverticulitis, and other gastrointestinal disorders. You don't need to supplement with 'prebiotics' if you eat fruits and vegetables.

Another benefit of fruits and vegetables is their ability to improve cognitive function and mental well-being. Studies have shown that consuming a diet high in fruits and vegetables is associated with a lower risk of cognitive decline and dementia. Additionally, these foods can improve mood and reduce symptoms of depression and anxiety.

They are also beneficial for the skin. They contain Vitamin C, which helps in the production of collagen. Collagen helps keep the skin firm, smooth, and elastic. They also contain carotenoids and flavonoids, which protect the skin from sun damage and UV rays.

Lastly, low glycemic fruits and vegetables are low in calories, making them an excellent choice for weight loss and weight management. They are also satisfying and can help reduce cravings and curb overeating.

CARBOHYDRATES OR CRACK?

My first job out of naturopathic medical school was detoxing drug addicts from cocaine, methamphetamines, heroin, alcohol, nicotine, methadone, etc. In my years of practice, I have delved into the fascinating world of the various substances humans become addicted to and their effects on the human body. My clinical experience mirrors medical research, and from my observation, carbohydrates are more addictive than cocaine. This may not surprise you if one of your ways of managing your life and emotions is to eat emotionally, and you feel like you are the victim of powerful carb cravings. Scientific research spanning several decades supports the fact that starches are not only delicious but also highly addictive.

However, carbohydrates, as a macronutrient, furnish the body with the energy it requires to perform its myriad functions. Found in foods like bread, pasta, rice, and potatoes, carbohydrates are almost immediately metabolized into glucose, which then fuels the body. Not all carbohydrates are created equal; simple carbohydrates, such as sugar, are readily absorbed by the body, causing a swift surge in blood sugar levels.

Spikes in blood sugar stimulate the release of dopamine, a neurotransmitter linked to pleasure and reward. Conventional nutritionists and carb lovers making excuses can say that complex carbohydrates are better, but they are like smoking a cigarette with a longer filter for a carb addict; not much different and still feeding the addiction.

If you want to lose weight, cut out sugars, grains, and starches. Even people doing high-intensity exercise don't need grains and simple sugars. Yams and sweet potatoes are the starches that savvy elite athletes choose most often. Want to know what a high rice intake gets you? The body of a sumo wrestler.

Dopamine is a crucial player in the brain's reward system, which spurs us to engage in activities essential for survival, like eating, avoiding predators, and procreation. When we undertake these activities, our brains unleash dopamine, making us feel gratified, reinforcing that behavior, and laying down pathways that become stronger the more we use them. This explains why we are naturally drawn to foods high in sugar and carbohydrates; they activate the reward system in our brains, eliciting euphoria and creating a positive feedback loop where the more sugar and carbohydrates we consume, the more dopamine is released, and the more we crave them.

This addiction can manifest in several ways, including cravings for sweet or starchy foods, difficulty controlling the amount of sugar and carbohydrates consumed, and withdrawal symptoms when cutting back. Some studies have even suggested that sugar addiction may be similar to drug addiction, with similar neural pathways and brain changes. The neurological effects of carbohydrate addiction are amplified when combined with neuroexcitatory additives like MSG and artificial colors.

Research has shown that sugar triggers the same brain regions as cocaine and other addictive drugs. For instance, a study conducted at the University of Bordeaux in France found that rats with unrestricted access to a sugary drink became addicted and continued to consume it even when given electric shocks. The researchers concluded that the rats had developed a dependence on sugar akin to drug addiction.

Another study from the University of Florida revealed that excessive sugar consumption can lead to modifications in the brain's reward system, resembling those seen in drug addiction. The researchers found that rats given high amounts of sugar suffered withdrawal symptoms when the sugar was withdrawn, including anxiety and depression. This may be why so many people eat emotionally and then get stuck in that habit.

These studies illustrate the addictive nature of

carbohydrates. While addiction is conventionally linked to drugs, alcohol, porn, gambling, shopping, and the media, it is evident that carbohydrates can also be highly addictive and can cause a host of chronic diseases.

I don't aim to suck the fun out of everything, as I am a foodie, after all. I love to eat fine food and have found that fresh, vital, healthy food is much more pleasing to the plate than your average American fare. I confess I am a bougie foodie, and while my smoothies only cost about $15 each compared to Gwyneth's $50 concoctions, I craft them in a way that would make the father of medicine proud.

"Let food be thy medicine and medicine be thy food."
~Hippocrates

I am asking for you to be mindful of the carbohydrates that you eat and avoid the ones that harpoon your health... or at least avoid them most of the time.

If you choose to eat them, only do so on special occasions. Birthdays, anniversaries, and holidays are good "cheat" days to have some delicious, starchy treats. But choose wisely. Do you crave a chocolate brownie? Or deserve a couple of glasses of wine? Or do you want to waste those carbs and calories on a basket of dinner rolls? Read your food labels and avoid foods with added sugars, and more carbs than protein.

EARN YOUR CARBS: BREAD, PASTA, POPCORN, ICE CREAM, WINE ETC

Carbohydrates have long been touted as the body's primary source of energy. However, the human body is a remarkable machine capable of utilizing various macronutrients for fuel. Fats and proteins can also be broken down into energy, making them viable alternatives to carbohydrates. You don't need carbohydrates in the amount you likely consume them, but they sure are delicious.

But what does 'earning your carbs' mean, exactly? It means you should actively burn the calories you consume through physical activity. If you're sedentary and consume high amounts of carbohydrates, your body is primed for prediabetes, weight gain, and chronic health issues from rampant inflammation and elevated blood sugar. Remember, high blood sugar is like broken glass pumping through your blood vessels, causing damage and a higher likelihood of heart attack, stroke, and dementia.

When you consume carbohydrates, your digestive system breaks them down into simple sugars, such as glucose, which are absorbed into the bloodstream. From there, insulin, a hormone produced by the pancreas, signals the body's cells to take up glucose and use it for energy or store it for later use.

However, if we consume more carbohydrates than our bodies need and are not engaging in physical activity to burn off the excess glucose, the body will store it as fat. This is because glucose is converted into glycogen, which is stored in the liver and muscles for future use. When these stores are full, excess glucose is converted into fat and stored in adipose tissue, leading to weight gain and other health problems.

Furthermore, chronically high blood sugar levels lead to insulin resistance, which can progress to type 2 diabetes and metabolic syndrome. In insulin resistance, the body's cells become less responsive to the effects of insulin, making it more difficult for glucose to enter the cells and be used for energy. As a result, glucose levels in the bloodstream remain elevated, leading to further complications, including heart disease, hormone imbalances, dementia, and cancer.

So, the next time you're about to indulge in a carb-heavy meal, ask yourself, *"Have I earned this? Is this meal in my best interest? Am I just eating for comfort or to stuff my emotions? Do I truly 'deserve' this fleeting sugar bomb of deliciousness?"* If not, consider going for a jog or hitting the gym before indulging, because these exercises will support your body rather than sabotage it. And remember, earning your carbs isn't about depriving yourself of the foods you love; it's about maintaining a healthy balance between diet and exercise. By doing so, you'll be on your way to a happier and healthier you.

Keep in mind, however, that no matter how much exercise you do, you won't be completely insulated from the negative health effects if you continue to eat like an irresponsible asshole.

"Let us bust the myth of physical inactivity and obesity. You cannot outrun a bad diet."
~Editorial in the British Medical Journal

RULE #4: FATS ARE YOUR FRIEND

Fats have a bad reputation, but in reality, they are essential. They provide energy, help absorb fat-soluble vitamins, and support the health of the brain, immune system, skin, and heart. Certain types of fats, such as monounsaturated and polyunsaturated fats, offer a wide range of health benefits. Monounsaturated fats, such as those found in olive oil, avocado, and nuts, have been shown to lower LDL cholesterol levels (the 'bad' cholesterol) and reduce the risk of heart disease. They also have anti-inflammatory properties, which can help reduce the risk of chronic diseases such as cancer, Alzheimer's disease, and Type 2 diabetes.

Polyunsaturated fats, such as those found in fatty fish like wild salmon, mackerel, sardines, seeds, and nuts, are particularly rich in omega-3 fatty acids. Omega-3 fatty acids improve heart health by reducing inflammation, triglycerides (a type of fat in the blood), and blood pressure. They also boost brain function, improve mood and cognitive function, and reduce the risk of depression and anxiety.

Saturated fats, typically found in animal products such as meat and dairy, have been linked to an increased risk of heart disease when consumed in excess. However, it's important to note that not all saturated fats are bad for health; some saturated fats, like those found in coconut oil, can have health benefits when consumed in moderate amounts. You can check your genetics to see if you are sensitive to saturated fats and would genuinely benefit from avoiding them.

As I said before, fats are an essential part of a healthy diet and can provide several health benefits. These include reducing the risk of heart disease, improving brain function, and reducing the risk of chronic diseases. However, it's important to be mindful of the types of fats you consume and to limit or avoid saturated and trans fats, which have been linked to an increased risk of chronic health conditions. Also, be sure to buy your dietary fats in glass containers rather than plastic. Many chemicals are lyophilic and can leach into the fats, which you then consume.

RULE #5: HIGH PROTEIN FOR STRUCTURE AND FUNCTION

Your DNA becomes you by creating the proteins that are the basis of your body's structure and how it functions. Proteins are made up of amino acids, which are the building blocks of basically everything. Proteins play a vital role in many bodily functions, such as hormone regulation, enzyme production, and maintaining a healthy immune system.

One of the main benefits of high-protein diets is weight loss. Proteins are more satisfying than carbohydrates or fats; they help reduce cravings and curb overeating. Additionally, proteins can boost metabolism, meaning the body burns more calories throughout the day.

Another benefit of high-protein diets is muscle building. Proteins are the primary building blocks of muscle tissue, and consuming enough protein can help promote muscle growth and repair. This is especially important for individuals who engage in regular strength-training exercises.

High-protein diets have also been shown to improve blood sugar control, which can benefit those with diabetes or those at risk of developing diabetes. Proteins can slow down digestion and the absorption of carbohydrates, which can help stabilize blood sugar levels. Proteins are also essential for the maintenance and repair of bones, and a diet rich in proteins can help prevent osteoporosis.

I recommend that my clients eat 100-200g of

protein per day, depending on their weight, activity level, and kidney function.

RULE #6: DON'T SKIP ON QUALITY

Be sure your protein sources are clean and high-quality. Quality options include organic grass-fed beef and dairy, wild-caught fish, organic pasture-raised or free-range organic chicken, and pasture-raised eggs. These foods are rich in essential amino acids, which are the building blocks of everything in your body. Non-organic meats, poultry, dairy, and farmed fish are full of toxins that build up in your body and harm your health.

RULE #7: AVOID PROCESSED FOODS

Food-like substances that come in boxes and bags aren't food. Avoid sugary, carbonated drinks and anything that has fake sugars. These foods are often high in calories or packed with artificial sweeteners. In fact, not only are they low in nutrients, but they are also contaminated with chemicals, artificial colors, preservatives, and other additives that contribute to weight gain, cancer, brain damage, hormone imbalances, and more.

Artificial colors are widely used in the food industry, but recent studies have raised concerns about the potential health risks associated with these synthetic dyes. These risks include cancer, hyperactivity and other behavioral problems in children, allergic reactions, and other health problems. To protect yourself, try to avoid artificial colors by choosing whole, unprocessed foods and reading ingredient labels. By being aware of the potential dangers, you can make informed choices and take control of your health.

Similarly, food preservatives are commonly added to foods to prolong their shelf life and prevent spoilage, but they have been linked to several negative health impacts. Cancer, allergic reactions, digestive disorders, and mental health conditions are a few of these. By choosing complete, unprocessed foods and carefully reading ingredient labels, you can try to protect yourself by avoiding food preservatives.

In my opinion, the Yuka app is a good resource for buying packaged foods because it can educate you about the health impacts of artificial flavors, colors, preservatives, etc. It doesn't consider carbohydrate content and isn't perfect, but it is a good place to start if you just can't stop eating cheesy crackers.

I use it to shop with my son. He can choose groceries that are in the green. Go ahead, use the app to scan your favorite snack food, read what the ingredients do to your health, and then decide if you really want to keep eating them.

The best medical interventions are subtractive, when you stop doing something that is harming your health. Not eating foods that poison you is a powerful first step toward wellness.

You are what you eat; nutrition serves as the cornerstone of optimal health and wellness. I've shared throughout this chapter my recommendations and supporting evidence for how the foods you choose to nourish your body directly influence your physical, mental, and emotional well-being. A balanced diet rich in essential nutrients, vitamins, and minerals is essential for maintaining the body's intricate systems and supporting its natural healing capabilities.

Conventional nutritionists create hospital food and

allow steak dinners after triple bypass surgery. A recent study showed that you can get all of your nutritional needs met with highly processed foods. I've had gastroenterologists and oncologists tell my patients that *"diet doesn't matter."* At these moments, I wish providers demonstrating willful stupidity were punished more immediately.

With a scientific and agenda-free understanding of human metabolism and the significance of micronutrients like vitamins and minerals, you gain the power to make informed choices about your diet. The synergistic effects of these nutrients work together to fortify our immune system, detox your body, support healthy digestion, and regulate vital functions like your heartbeat, hormone production, and neurotransmitters.

Your food choices play a crucial role in preventing chronic diseases and promoting longevity. By embracing whole, unprocessed foods and minimizing the consumption of artificial additives and excessive carbohydrates and sugars, you empower your body to thrive.

CHAPTER 14
MYA

Moving your body is an excellent treatment for basically everything that can go wrong with your health.　　ALMOST　　EVERYTHING! (99.999999999999% of things) such as dementia, diabetes, heart disease, cancer, pain, autoimmune diseases, anxiety, depression, fibromyalgia, insomnia, MS, digestive issues, lack of self-esteem, fatigue, hating your life, bad relationships, acne, irritability, infertility, hormone imbalances, headaches, etc. Well, if you overexercise, that is a whole other problem that exercise itself cannot fix. But exercise based on anorexia is really the only thing exercise won't improve. But then what about everything else?

We have research showing that exercise improves outcomes, progression, and quality of life. It is super badass all around. I don't want to overuse the word 'exercise,' as I know that no one wants another 'exercise' lecture. It's overdone. Let's call it something else.　　Joyful　　movement?　　Too　　hippy-dippy. Calisthenics? Nope, we aren't 80 years old. From here on out, the activity formerly known as 'exercise' will now be referred to as *Moving Your Ass (MYA)*.

According to the CDC, you are most likely one of the 80% of people who know they aren't MYA as much as recommended. Now, please allow me to channel the bitch goddess of victory, Nike: *"Just fucking do it. Move your ass!"* First, I have a question for you. What is holding you back? Be honest!

For you nerds who need some science to decide that exercise is good for you, here are my top 10 physiologic benefits of MYA:

PHYSIOLOGICAL BENEFITS OF MYA

1. More muscle, increased strength, and healthier bones. Let me spell it out for you. More muscle means stronger bones, so you can avoid osteoporosis—aka brittle bones. You want to decrease your likelihood of having brittle bones because weak bones mean a much higher chance of breaking your hip as you age. If you break your hip, you are up to 37% more likely to die in the next year and 75% more likely to be institutionalized in a nursing home because you don't heal well enough to be autonomous.

2. Increased blood flow and improved cardiovascular health mean better healing and a decreased likelihood of heart attacks and strokes.

3. Sweating helps you detoxify nasty toxicants from your body and improves your skin's health. Yep, it makes you glow and decreases acne and breakouts.

4. Increases your energy levels and decreases pain.

5. Increases endorphins for mental health and can make you feel happier. It also decreases your likelihood of getting dementia and ending up in a nursing home.

6. Decreases your risk of getting chronic diseases like diabetes. Diabetes can cause you to go blind and lose your limbs... and, you guessed it, end up in a nursing home.

7. Improves sleep.

8. Improves sex life.

9. Improves your microbiome and optimizes your immune system's function.

10. It makes you look better in hot pants, giving you better options for your sex life.

But you probably already knew that.

WHAT ARE YOUR EXCUSES FOR NOT MYA?

Are you in pain or hurt? MYA is good for chronic pain. I didn't just make that up. You can Google it. Also, that is why people go to physical therapists. If you have an injury, get an excellent personal trainer and/or a physical therapist and learn how to move to support the healing of your injury.

Are you tired? MYA is proven to decrease stress and increase energy levels. You just have to get up and do it. Nothing is in your way except for the excuses you make for yourself and the obstacles you place in front of your greatness. So quit that shit! I don't even really care about what you do for MYA, but I promise that when you commit to doing it, your whole life will be better.

You cannot be healthy if you sit all day. You may starve yourself, so you are skinny-fat (you are skinny but don't have healthy muscle), and your body fat is higher than that of a healthy body. You may look okay, but your body won't feel okay for long because it was made to move. It needs to move. Unleash your inner tigress/stallion with more than just tequila.

MYA isn't about weight loss. Weight loss is so much more complicated than just calories in vs. calories out. Moving your body and feeling like a bad ass gladiator bitch in love with your skin is the primary goal for you. When you move your body with joy and laughter, when you smile and get down into your skin, bones, and muscles in a concerted and present way, you blow open your mind and your body's receptors and give your general health a big bolus of awesomeness. Guess what? You become healthier and happier by making micro-movements in all the health categories we discuss.

Remember: When you are gentle with yourself yet committed to your optimal well-being, you will most likely achieve your optimal size, shape, and weight, the weight that is healthy for you. But the more you worry about your weight, the less likely you are to lose it because of stress hormones. So, give up on the stress. You are beautiful. You are loveable, and you can still make choices that improve your health.

Do you want to be strong, healthy, and happy? Move. Do it for that reason, not because someone else thinks you should be wearing smaller pants.

On the other hand, however, I would be remiss if I did not say that having too much fat on your body in the wrong places is dangerous and unhealthy. Do I want you to be gloriously healthy, happy, and wise? YES!

Do I think everyone should weigh 120 lbs? Hell, No. Healthy comes in all shapes and sizes, but morbidly obese isn't one of them.

EXERCISE IDEAS

• **Love to Dance?** Twerk your ass or get on a pole in a stripper class. Put on a playlist and dance in your underwear. It isn't a cliché! It is a way of enjoying your body and showing off how you have moves that Beyoncé and Lizzo could be jealous of.

• **Love your dog?** Walk it. Don't just take it to a dog park and sit and watch it run. Move with the dog. Guess what? MYA is good for both of you.

- **Love sex?** Sex is exercise! Don't just lay there; use this time as an opportunity to get your squats, planks, and pushups while enjoying a pleasurable experience. Try out new positions. Get the Kama Sutra out of the library. Put on a sexy playlist and make it a workout (please practice safe sex—physically, mentally, and emotionally).

- **Are you a little bit OCD and love order?** Ha! Cleaning is an excellent way to MYA. Get out a sponge, stay away from the nasty cleaners, and use your elbow grease. My favorite are the eraser sponges, which work like chelators for dirt! I love science. Don't forget to choose biodegradable, natural cleaners like vinegar and baking soda to clean the house!

- **Love to chill and lay around?** Do yoga! There are three million ways to do yoga within a mile of you right now. Pick one. Yoga is awesome. There are plenty of voluptuous and gorgeous yogis on Instagram to follow. You can join me for *Lazy Bitch Yoga,* which I sporadically Livestream on Facebook and Instagram. Yoga is a stress buster, a flexibility improver (mentally, physically, and emotionally), and a muscle strengthener.

- **Lift Weights.** Yes, groceries and children count. Don't get all crazy about cardio; it can be more stressful on your body and can further imbalance your hormones. My favorite exercise programs are all about weights, and for good reasons. You can increase your heart rate and build more muscle, which is highly metabolic. Muscle cells burn calories just by existing.

Working a muscle group to failure (meaning you can't possibly do even one more pushup or bicep curl) completely resets the muscle's sensitivity to insulin. Insulin resistance is a health crisis in this country and leads to Type II diabetes, metabolic syndrome, PCOS, heart disease, obesity, and fuels cancer and dementia. Kettlebell workouts are my go-to exercise, and I travel with exercise bands. Bodyweight exercises and workouts are all you need to get started on a fitness journey. Squats, pushups, lunges, and abdominal exercises work the major muscle groups of the body and need no equipment.

• **Go Swimming.** My favorite things to do in water are skinny dipping and lying around in hot springs. However, that doesn't count as exercise. I love to swim; the quiet and the metered breathing are deeply meditative for me. I am not a huge fan of chlorine because it can impair your thyroid function, so I choose saltwater pools whenever possible. Swimming is excellent for strength, breathing, and cardio and can be preferable if you have sore joints from high-impact sports or have spent too much time on your knees in college.

• **Go Hiking.** I like to get outside and climb mountains whenever I can. You get sunshine, vitamin D, vitamin N (from nature, and it is proven to be fantastic for you), fresh air, and exercise all at the same time! It is health multitasking at its finest. Hiking is especially excellent because you often go places where you don't have cell service and can disconnect from the world.

• **Try Something New.** Tennis, beach volleyball, basketball, golf, pickleball... who cares? Explore Orange Theory, Curves, Barre, Bikram, Silver Sneakers, Pilates, or Salsa. Whatever your jam is, please just do it with joy and appreciate your body for the superb vehicle it is.

Patients often ask me: *"What is the best kind of exercise?"* The answer is, *"The kind you do."*

TIPS FOR MYA SUCCESS

- **Start slow:** Many fitness gurus or programs don't appreciate or talk about easing your way into workout programs. They recommend jumping in at New Year's with gym memberships and running on the treadmill like you are following the first rule of the zombie apocalypse: Cardio. Then you can't walk the next day and don't get back into the gym until May because swimsuit season is coming. Easing into exercise decreases the likelihood of getting injured and creates success in the long term by cementing habits into your neurology.

- **Pay attention to your body:** Are you slouching with your shoulders rounded and your chin jutting forward? Do you have a 'nerd neck' from looking down at your phone, making it more likely that you will get a dowager's hump? Is your stomach pushed out, or is your core engaged? Are you breathing deeply or shallowly? Do you stand and sit up straight? Is your weight balanced equally on both legs and hips? How do you walk? With purpose and power? Do you shuffle and slouch, or do you sashay ole' like you own the world with loose, supple hips, a tight core, shoulders back, chin high, and a smile on your face? If you aren't used to it, having proper posture is a workout all in itself.

- **Workout Smart:** After paying attention to how you hold your body and posture, you may have identified that you favor one side of your body. It makes sense because most of us aren't ambidextrous, and many of us have had injuries to one side of our body that we unconsciously learned to compensate for.

When you are balanced on both sides of your body, injuries are less likely to occur. Remember, one of the secrets to beauty is symmetry. I like to do asymmetrical movements, so my strong side can't compensate for the weaker side. That is why I don't do machines and use free weights and bodyweight exercises more often. Machines stabilize for you, and while they will isolate muscles for more definition and specific rehab, the co-movers and stabilizers get to be lazy and not work as hard. Ugh, that just means you need to spend more time, MYA!

- **Change it up:** Exercise is best when it is varied and progressive. The body adapts to the same movements quickly anyway, decreasing effectiveness and fitness impact.

- **Make it fun:** If it isn't fun, you won't do it. Find something you like to do besides drink, swipe, binge TV, and trawl social media on your couch. Engage in life. Don't just let it pass you by.

- **Schedule it:** Put a reminder on your phone that dings with a pump-up song and hold yourself accountable. This works until you don't care about the reminder anymore. You let all your MYA motivation go to shit, so...

- **Be Accountable**: Find a partner to work out with, and make sure it is one who won't accept your excuses or flake out on you: Accountability is a powerful tool and is integral in supporting exercise and lifestyle changes. If you were internally motivated, you would most likely already have a successful workout program and an Instagram channel about it. But if you aren't, you are externally motivated, and well, that's okay. You just need more support, so find online communities, friends who need to move their asses, meetup groups, or hire a personal trainer. Stop making excuses. Just stop already.

> *"Do or do not. There is no try."*
> *~Master Yoda*

Are you telling yourself that you are too tired and depressed, too 'busy,' or too [INSERT YOUR EXCUSE HERE]? Change your attitude. Make yourself a priority, and make the time and commitment to exercise.

Prioritize your Health: Support yourself rather than sabotage. Decide that you are worth it. I want you to treat yo'self by committing to making yourself a priority, loving yourself to the bone, and doing the things that will nurture and sustain your health, wellness, power, joy, and happiness over the long term. Do not just treat yo'self to donuts, designer labels, and Botox. I want you to believe that you deserve the finest things in life and treat yo' self to body and soul, revolutionizing self-care and not meaningless shit that makes you obese, tired, sick, and in debt. No matter what culture and media tell you, materialism does not fill the insatiable hole of meaninglessness that still gapes inside of you.

Self-awareness, self-care, and self-love are the avenues to true joy and purpose. Authentic joy and purpose have the capacity to complete you... not Jerry Maguire. BARF. Motivate yourself with a carrot and a stick. Put a picture of an older person in a nursing home on your wall for some 'stick' motivation, or better yet, go inside and tour one of those hellholes. That will be a stellar motivator to remind yourself why

MYA is important. And choose your carrot—what do you really want to reward yourself with?

MYA is important—really freaking important. I implore you to motivate yourself not out of fear but rather out of love. Love yourself. MYA a little every day, in a meaningful way. Sweating, breathing a little heavy, and adding muscle to your body make it 1000 times more likely that you will live a long and healthy life. Choose wisely whether next time your first instinct is to be an exhausted, sedentary blob on the couch watching TV, eating fast food, and complaining your thyroid isn't working, or if you want to live a healthy life and enjoy it to the fullest. Remember, after all, exercise is good for your thyroid.

CHAPTER 15
INVEST IN SLEEP AND THRIVE

Chances are you aren't getting enough quality sleep, and that causes all kinds of harm to your mind and body. In a nutshell, sleep deprivation makes the likelihood of you dying from everything higher. My brothers and I tease our mother about her response when we were kids and we complained about anything and everything.

"Mom, I have a headache."

"Mom, I have a stomachache."

"Mom, I don't feel good."

"Mom, I have a broken leg."

Her answer was simply, *"Go to bed."*

She has always been ahead of her time.

You may not think you are sleep-deprived, but getting less than 7 hours of quality sleep a night can lead to:

- Hypertension, heart disease, and stroke
- Weight gain, obesity, and type II Diabetes
- Depression, anxiety, and psychiatric disorders
- Memory loss, problems with mood and attention
- Decreased critical thinking and creativity
- Decreased fertility and low sex drive
- Impaired immune function
- Memory loss, irritability, and brain shrinkage
- Increased likelihood of accidents

- Being a bitch and not the good kind that is Babe (or Bro) in total control of Her(or Him)self.

We spend about one-third of our lives sleeping. However, there is a vast difference between lying in bed with your eyes closed and having good quality sleep. I love my fitness tracker because, while it may not be perfectly accurate, it helps hold me accountable to go to bed on time and indicates whether I am getting good sleep or tossing and turning all night. I am also able to see the results of my daily routines and behaviors and whether my sleep is improved by taking certain supplements, working out more, etc.

SLEEP AND YOUR BRAIN

Sleep affects everything, and it is especially vital to brain health. Sleep impacts several brain functions, including how nerve cells (neurons) communicate with each other. In fact, during sleep, our brain stays remarkably active. Sleep is an essential aspect of overall health and has a direct impact on brain function.

- **Memory Consolidation:** Sleep helps to solidify and integrate new information into existing knowledge structures, which is essential for learning and memory. Sleep also plays a role in the formation of long-term memories.

- **Cognitive Function:** Sleep has been shown to improve cognitive abilities, including attention, concentration, and problem-solving. A lack of sleep can impair these functions, making it more difficult to complete tasks and make decisions.

- **Mood Regulation:** Sleep has a significant impact on mood, with chronic sleep deprivation leading to an increased risk of depression and anxiety. Adequate sleep has been shown to improve mood and reduce symptoms of depression and anxiety.

- **Neuroprotection:** Sleep has been shown to play a role in the removal of waste products from the brain, including the clearance of neurotoxins that can contribute to neurodegenerative diseases such as Alzheimer's.

Fun fact: sleeping on your side helps detoxify your brain better. Back sleep is second best, and if you sleep on your stomach, uh oh! It would serve to retrain yourself to sleep on your back or side.

I have an entrepreneur client who thought sleep was unnecessary. His motto was that he'd sleep when he was dead. He ended up decimating his immune system and getting cardiomegaly, splenomegaly, and hepatomegaly from inflammation and chronic viral infections because his body was too weary to mount a response. He started sleeping and managing stress by meditating, long walks on the beach – no kidding- and everything improved and resolved. He completely overhauled his life and is much happier and healthier. Make sleep a priority!

AMPLIFY YOUR SLEEP

Let's concentrate on improving the sleep you have. These are fundamental rules to follow if you want to overhaul your sleep patterns.

1. Turn Your Bedroom into a Sleepy Sex Palace: Your bedroom is your lair. Make it a holy place for your sexiness. Beauty is bone-deep, not skin-deep. If you aren't healthy, you aren't hot. I don't care how many hair extensions, push-up bras, Spanx, fake eyelashes, and makeup contouring methods you employ, that shit will eventually come off. You need sleep to be sexy.

2. No TV. No phone. No screens: You should only do two things in bed—sleep and sex—nothing else. Program your brain to expect one of two glorious things, so it isn't confused about what is going on. Screens emit blue light, which tells your brain that it is daytime and not time to sleep.

If you watch TV or use your phone or tablet after dark because you don't live in the freaking stone age of the 1980s, get blue-blocker glasses. I prefer the type with amber lenses because they seem to work better for me – I get sleepier faster when I read. If you wear glasses to read, try these. Meow!

3. Luxurious bed: Make your bed into a luxurious nest with sheets and blankets that make you feel like a queen, a Khaleesi, or an intergalactic star lord. I have silk pillowcases that make my heart sing. They are gentle on your skin and hair, feel glorious, and are made of natural fibers, so they don't emit microplastics into the environment. I gave everyone in my family some as gifts one year. They are an inexpensive luxury that you can enjoy every day. Get some colors that make you feel glorious and add to your sexy boudoir or sleepy cave environment.

Heavy weighted blankets can help you feel more calm and secure, like swaddling a fussy baby. If you have elevated stress hormones that make your sleep difficult, this may be a helpful option for you:

Try to get natural fibers so you don't poison yourself or the water. These are more difficult to find and made entirely of natural fibers, so try other interventions before this one. Many of these sorts of items have some polyester and aren't organic cotton, but you must pick your freaking battles, right? Better sleep? Yes. A weighted blanket made by a well-paid indigenous person from recycled paper and free-range silkworms isn't something you can easily find in most places, yet, so do your best. It will all be okay. We don't need to have a nervous breakdown about being perfect. Right? Just let some of that shit go.

4. Decrease Sensory Stimulation: Are you a parent tuned to every noise in the night, making sure your precious angel doesn't stop breathing or burn the house down? Are you a naturally light sleeper? Invest in earplugs and an eye mask. I use an eye mask to block light and earplugs, so I don't have to listen to the farting and snoring of my... dog.

Blackout shades may also be extremely helpful if you are light-sensitive. Human nature is to wake with the sun, and this is especially troublesome if you work the night shift. Having a disrupted circadian rhythm is disastrous for health.

Light exposure affects the release of hormones such as melatonin and cortisol, which can affect sleep and wake cycles, mood, and alertness. By blocking out light, blackout shades can help improve the quality and duration of sleep, leading to a more regulated release of neurotransmitters and improved overall brain function.

5. Keep your room cool, filter your bedroom air, and get some white noise: The optimal temperature for sleeping is about 65°F. Check out this bed cooler – It blows air at your desired temperature to cool hot sleepers. Since you probably don't live in the Himalayas or the Alps, you should be filtering the air in your bedroom anyway. The Austin Air Filter is the best system I know of, recommended by most doctors specializing in environmental medicine. It acts as a fan and can be loud AF in its highest setting – so it also supplies white noise. My son has had one in his bedroom since he was born, because we live in a city with less than awesome air quality. I remember TV commercials from my childhood in the 1980s that connected poor air quality and asthma. Instead of protecting and cleaning the air, prescriptions for allergy medications and inhalers were much simpler and lucrative to implement. Knowledge is power, and so I also have this model, which helped protected us from the poor air quality during the California fires. Are you going to choose to protect yourself and your family with this information? I hope so.

6. Get a New Bed: Does your bed suck? Are you uncomfortable when you sleep? Explore other options if you need a new mattress. Go with natural fibers and options to find one that suits your sleeping preferences and doesn't poison you. Many memory foam options off-gas chemicals for months, which add to your toxic body burden and lead to migraines, cancer, obesity, and other chronic diseases.

7. Establish a Soothing Pre-Sleep Routine: Routines help the brain recognize a pattern and settle into a comfortable habit and behavior. The more you practice something, the stronger the neural pathways supporting it become, making it second nature—a habit.

For many of us, our days are full of stressful situations, irritation, bullshit, responsibility, drama, #adulting, and angst, even if it is just the TV show you watch at the end of the evening. Signaling the body to start relaxing and getting ready for sleep is part of good sleep hygiene and supports sleep success. You can begin about an hour before bed and slow your roll.

Here are some ideas to support your best sleep:

Take a bath: Hot Epsom salt baths are a great way to relax your body and get extra magnesium for neurotransmitter production. They are also remarkably detoxifying and can help lower higher levels of stress hormones that can make deep, regenerative sleep difficult.

Read a book: I mean a real book; one with pages. Remember those? They don't have the blue light of screens and can help your brain wind down and relax. Read some organic chemistry, which always did it for me in college.

Practice relaxation exercises: YouTube has a billion hypnosis techniques, binaural beats, music, meditations, white noise, etc., for sleep. Try some and see. Meditation and hypnosis are powerful tools to support sleep. If it doesn't work the first time, try again. Creating new neural pathways takes practice and repetition for them to become more powerful habits than those you have been doing for the last 20 years.

Avoid stress: Avoid doing stressful and stimulating activities, such as working, violent TV or video games, or discussing emotional issues. Don't bring your work home; stop checking your emails at all hours and give yourself downtime to enjoy the part of your life that isn't about work.

Doing physically and psychologically stressful activities can cause the body to produce cortisol (the stress hormone), which is associated with increased alertness. If you think this is an issue for you, try a sleep supplement to decrease your cortisol and improve your sleep.

Do some light activity before bed: You don't want to do cardio before bed because it can raise your endorphin levels, but gentle bodyweight exercises can increase growth hormone production and support healthy sleep. Don't go nuts and get all swol', but some bodyweight squats before bed, a few push-ups, and lunges can support sleep. Having sex or doing night yoga are other great options to prepare for bed.

No late-night snacking: Be aware of the impact that late night snacking has on sleep quality. If you crave carbs at night, you are likely eating them to produce more serotonin, a relaxing neurotransmitter.

Snacking before bed can affect sleep quality in different ways, depending on the type and amount of food consumed. Consuming a light, healthy snack that contains a small amount of carbohydrate and protein, especially tryptophan (an amino acid found in foods like turkey, milk, and bananas), can help promote sleep by increasing serotonin levels, which is a neurotransmitter that helps regulate sleep. On the other hand, consuming a heavy, high-fat snack close to bedtime can cause indigestion and disrupt sleep as the body is focused on digestion instead of rest.

Chocolate is high in magnesium, another ingredient that supports serotonin production. You can get your neurotransmitters tested and see how they can be supported naturally rather than risking adding more lbs. to your waist with "bon bon" therapy. Because if you aren't sleeping, you aren't losing weight. Sleep is one of the significant factors in weight loss that isn't usually addressed.

Explore the effect of food on your sleep and see what your body likes best. I have a client who stops eating at 6pm and now sleeps better than ever.

Avoid Intake of Caffeine, Nicotine, and Other Stimulants: Know what increases cortisol levels in your body? Caffeine. Yep. So only have it in the morning, especially if you have trouble sleeping. Nicotine can also be stimulatory for the brain, and smokers should refrain from using tobacco products too close to their scheduled bedtime. Attention medications and other drugs can also impact sleep.

Avoid Alcohol: Alcohol is known to promote "sleep" after consumption. However, we all know it begins to act like a stimulant after a few hours of Irish Car Bombs and tequila shots. Our sleep, after a bender, gets shittier with increased awakenings and decreased overall sleep quality as we get older.

Increasing your bifidobacterial (probiotic), liver cleanse supplements, plenty of water, and B vitamins can help with hangovers. Feeling like ass after drinking is a combination of dehydration and nutrient depletion. Your neurotransmitters take a hit, and your liver isn't as spry as it used to be. So, to avoid this, take your supplements, hydrate, and your hangovers will be non-existent if you do choose to drink. Unfortunately, those supplements won't do much for the extra calories and weight gain from alcoholic drinks.

Functional Medicine and Testing: Testing your hormones, food sensitivities, and neurotransmitters at NaturopathicMD.com can give you vital information on many different aspects of your health, not just sleep. You can also order supplements to support healthy sleep patterns and decrease the adverse effects of not sleeping well.

Hormones have a huge role in sleep. The first symptoms of perimenopause often begin when progesterone levels drop in relation to estrogen, and the imbalance leads to sleep disruption, hot flashes, anxiety, and weight gain.

If you are experiencing any of these, the hormonal aspects can be addressed naturally by supporting progesterone production or using an over-the-counter cream. Bioidentical hormone replacement has a time and place, so don't rule that out in the future, either. Contact me with questions about Bioidentical Hormone Replacement and recommendations for the best kind of providers. If it isn't done well, it can be dangerous.

Food sensitivities can increase histamine and endorphins in the brain (which are stimulating neurotransmitters) and make sleep difficult. Neurotransmitter levels can be optimized to promote sleep as well.

Everyone is different, and no one knows exactly why we sleep, how much is best to get, or when to exercise, eat, etc., to optimize it. Just like almost everything else, the answer is probably personalized and some variation of *"It depends."*

I don't claim to be an expert on your sleep. My goal is for you to become an expert in your sleep by implementing different testing, activities, and interventions, tracking your experience and success, and making changes that help you get out of bed in the morning with energy, gusto, and a positive attitude so you can Live Your Best Life.

CHAPTER 16
DETOX YOUR HOME BY CHOOSING CLEAN PRODUCTS

Avoiding harmful chemicals in the first place decreases how much exposure you have. Decreasing your exposure means you have less toxicants in your body (or bucket) and how often you need to detoxify or open up the spigot for your body to feel well.

I recently wrote a research document with over fifty pages and almost five hundred clinical research references for a medical testing company that looks at chemical exposures in humans. My findings were that you are exposed to massive amounts of chemicals through breathing, eating, drinking, and your skin, which are known to disrupt your health.

I've been having trouble communicating this next section because the terrain is always changing. If you follow me on social media, you will see examples of products that used to be clean and non-toxic when they were owned and managed by the founders, who were passionate about non-toxic products. We all know that once the company is bought, the packaging doesn't have to change except for the new owners being added to the back of the label. But unfortunately, I think that companies like Unilever don't give a fuck about having clean and non-toxic products that they made in the past because they know that they can charge more for the toxic products they are making now.

Unfortunately, while you weren't obsessively reading the labels of your favorite products because you remember it was created by a Grandma who donates profits to the third world and you trusted them, they changed the formula, and now it contains poisonous shit!

I'm a pretty mellow person; I go with the flow most of the time, but this is one of my hot buttons. I am big on trust, and I don't want to recommend certain products and companies to you when ingredients change all the time. It will serve you to know what you are looking for on labels and check in now and then. A product that says it is 'natural and paraben-free' can still have artificial fragrance and other toxicants in it. The situation is a lot like 'BPA-free' and 'fructose' because companies know consumers are getting savvy, and so they find loopholes—those rat bastards.

In my opinion, the most effective way of voting is with your purchases, and I get really pissed when I pay $11 for a deodorant that isn't as clean as the marketing says. My partner bought me some luxurious bath salts with rose petals in them. He knows I'm very conscious of all the products I buy and use, and so he did what he thought was due diligence when shopping for them. It said it was 'vegan, paraben-free, and gluten-free,' but it still had toxic 'fragrance' and harmful colorings in it. The FDA makes it possible for the 'organic' label to be used on food products that have 5% or less non-organic ingredients. The European Union prohibits or significantly limits 1600 chemicals in personal care products; the FDA only prohibits nine. Do you think the US government has your best interest in mind?

So, who do you trust? It depends on educating yourself and being your own advocate. Read labels because companies regularly acquire and change ingredients. I post about different products I like on social media and offer a webinar where I share my most up-to-date resources and educate you about how to purchase the best products for you and your family.

Here are some general recommendations for chemicals to avoid, and you can go step by step, room by room, to detoxify your home and make it a healthier place for you and those you love.

Yuka is an app that I like for cleaning and personal care products; it is also pretty good for food. I like to cross-reference it with resources at ewg.org because they keep up with the research.

HOUSEHOLD PRODUCTS

Forever chemicals, also known as per- and poly-fluoroalkyl substances (PFAS), are a group of human-made chemicals that are commonly found in household products, including non-stick cookware, waterproof clothing, stain guard, food packaging, and even some cleaning products.

These chemicals are called 'forever' because they do not break down naturally in the environment and can persist in the environment and our bodies for years - even the detox I designed doesn't get them out very well. Research has linked exposure to PFAS to a wide range of health problems, including cancer, reproductive and developmental issues, immune system dysfunction, and thyroid disease. They can be absorbed easily through the digestive system and skin and bioaccumulate, so even low-level exposure to these chemicals builds up over time and causes health issues.

It's important to be aware of the products in your home that may contain PFAS and take steps to reduce your exposure. Look for products labeled as PFAS-free, avoid non-stick cookware, stay away from stain guards and water-proof fabrics, and opt for natural or organic cleaning products. If you have Teflon pans, throw them out even if they aren't scratched.

FABRICS

Common fire retardants used in clothing, such as PBDEs, chlorinated Tris, and antimony trioxide, have been linked to a variety of health issues. PBDEs, for example, have been associated with thyroid disruption, reproductive problems, and developmental issues in children. Chlorinated Tris has been classified as a probable human carcinogen and has also been associated with developmental problems.

While fire retardants may be effective at preventing fabrics from catching fire, they can have negative impacts on our health, especially with repeated exposure. So, when possible, it's best to choose clothing made from natural fibers like cotton, linen, wool, silk, etc., which are less likely to require fire retardants.

MICROPLASTICS

The largest source of microplastic pollution is the breakdown of larger plastic products, such as plastic bags, bottles, and packaging materials. Remember, plastic doesn't biodegrade back into the environment to be reused. When these larger plastics are exposed to sunlight, wind, and water, they begin to break down into smaller and smaller particles, eventually becoming microplastics.

These particles pose a threat to our environment, as they can be ingested by marine life and end up in our food chain. A massive source of microplastics comes from artificial fabrics like fleece, polyester, nylon, and acrylic. It is estimated that a single load of laundry can release 700,000 microplastic particles into our waterways. To reduce your exposure to microplastics in fabrics, choose natural materials like cotton, wool, silk, or linen. They are more expensive in the short term but will pay off later in health rewards.

In addition to their environmental impact, microplastics also have negative health effects; obviously, they can get into your bloodstream and even into your cells! Studies have shown that microplastics can accumulate in human tissues and organs, potentially leading to inflammation, oxidative stress, and even cancer. Microplastics can also disrupt our hormones and negatively affect our immune system, leading to a variety of health issues. *Gross.*

"Fuck plastic or plastic will fuck you."
~***Dr. Heather Wilde***

WHAT CAN YOU DO?

1. Change the way you purchase everything, and always choose non-plastic options when available.

2. Use reusable water bottles made of glass or stainless steel instead of disposable plastic bottles.

3. Use a refillable coffee cup instead of a disposable one. Even paper coffee cups are lined with plastic.

4. Use natural fiber clothing, such as cotton, linen, silk, and wool, instead of synthetic materials like polyester and nylon.

5. Attach a microplastic filter to reduce microfiber shedding, or wash clothes in a bag like GuppyFriend by Patagonia.

6. Avoid single-use plastic products like straws, utensils, and bags. Get reusable produce bags so you don't add to the plastic pollution that castrates our boys and hormone bombs our girls by inundating them with xenoestrogens.

7. Support companies that prioritize sustainable and eco-friendly practices.

8. Use a reusable grocery bag instead of a plastic one.

9. Support organizations that research and work to reduce plastic pollution.

10. Use non-plastic alternatives to household items, such as bamboo or metal utensils, instead of plastic ones.

11. Do not store your food in plastic.

12. Minimize eating takeout because we know those plastic chemicals in Styrofoam and other containers transfer easily to food.

13. Spread awareness about the issue and encourage others to take action to reduce plastic pollution. Support legislation that bans or regulates the use of plastics in consumer products. I'm pretty sure, like the tobacco companies, plastic companies have known all along what an environmental disaster and hormonal shitshow they have been contributing to for the last 50 years. Are you going to help hold them accountable?

INGREDIENTS TO AVOID IN PERSONAL CARE PRODUCTS AND COSMETICS:

- **Parabens:** These are preservatives commonly

found in cosmetics and personal care products that have been linked to endocrine disruption and breast cancer.

• **Phthalates:** These chemicals are often used in fragrances and have been linked to cancer, reproductive toxicity, and developmental problems.

• **Formaldehyde:** This is a known carcinogen and is often used as a preservative in cosmetics and hair straightening treatments.

• **Triclosan:** This is an antibacterial agent that has been linked to hormone disruption and can contribute to the development of antibiotic-resistant bacteria.

• **Sodium lauryl sulfate (SLS) and sodium laureth sulfate (SLES):** These are foaming agents commonly found in shampoos and body washes that can cause skin irritation and strip the skin of its natural oils.

• **Polyethylene glycols (PEGs):** These are synthetic chemicals often used as thickeners and can be contaminated with carcinogens such as ethylene oxide and 1,4-dioxane.

• **Synthetic fragrances:** These can contain dozens of potentially harmful chemicals that can trigger allergies, respiratory problems, and skin irritation.

• **Coal tar:** This is a known carcinogen and is often found in hair dyes and anti-dandruff shampoos.

• **Toluene:** This is a solvent commonly found in nail polish and has been linked to reproductive and developmental toxicity.

• **Mineral oil:** This is a petroleum-derived ingredient often used as a moisturizer, but it can clog pores and interfere with the skin's natural functions.

• **Hydroquinone:** This is a skin-lightening agent that has been linked to skin irritation, ochronosis (a blue-black discoloration of the skin), and even cancer.

• **Retinyl palmitate:** This is a form of vitamin A often found in anti-aging products but can increase the risk of skin cancer when exposed to sunlight.

• **Lead:** This is a heavy metal that can be found in some lipsticks and has been linked to neurotoxicity and developmental delays in children.

• **Aluminum:** This is a metal that is often found in antiperspirants and has been linked to breast cancer and Alzheimer's disease.

• **Talc:** This is a mineral that is often found in makeup products such as powder, eyeshadow, and blush and has been linked to ovarian cancer when used in the genital area. This has been used on babies for years!

• **BHA and BHT:** These are synthetic antioxidants often found in lipsticks and moisturizers that have been linked to cancer and endocrine disruption.

• **Propylene glycol:** This is a synthetic ingredient often used as a humectant and can cause skin irritation and allergic reactions.

• **Ethanolamines (MEA, DEA, and TEA):** These are chemicals used to adjust the pH of products and can cause skin irritation and allergic reactions.

• **Formaldehyde donors (DMDM hydantoin, imidazolidinyl urea, diazolidinyl urea):** These are preservatives that release formaldehyde over time and can cause skin irritation and allergic reactions.

• **Methylisothiazolinone (MI):** This is a preservative commonly found in personal care products that can cause skin irritation and allergic reactions.

• **Synthetic colors:** These are artificial dyes often found in makeup and hair products that can cause skin irritation and allergic reactions.

• **Sunscreen chemicals oxybenzone, octinoxate, octocrylene, and homosalate:** These are chemical sunscreen ingredients that have been linked to skin irritation, endocrine disruption, and coral reef damage.

• **Synthetic emulsifiers:** These are synthetic ingredients used to bind oil and water in cosmetics and can cause skin irritation and allergic reactions. Examples include: polysorbate 20, Polysorbate 80, PEG-40, Cetearyl alcohol, Glyceryl stearate, and Sodium lauryl sulfate.

INGREDIENTS TO AVOID IN HOUSEHOLD CLEANING PRODUCTS:

• **Triclosan:** This chemical is often found in antibacterial cleaning products and has been linked to potential hormone disruption, including thyroid hormone disruption, and may contribute to antibiotic resistance.

• **Phthalates:** These are a group of chemicals often used in cleaning products as fragrance ingredients and have been linked to potential hormone disruption, including reproductive and developmental problems.

• **Sodium Lauryl Sulfate (SLS):** This is a

foaming agent often found in cleaning products such as dish soap that can cause skin irritation and is linked to potential autoimmune diseases.

• **Formaldehyde:** This is a preservative often found in cleaning products that can be harmful if inhaled and is linked to potential cancer risks.

• **Ammonia:** This chemical is often found in glass cleaners and can irritate the eyes, skin, and respiratory system.

• **Chlorine bleach:** This chemical is often found in disinfectants and can cause skin and eye irritation and respiratory problems. It can also be harmful if ingested.

• **Glycol ethers, AKA Butyl glycol ether, Butoxyethanol, Ethylene glycol butyl ether, Butyl Oxitol, EGBE, Butyl cellosolve acetate (the acetate form):** These are solvents often used in cleaning products that can cause skin and eye irritation, respiratory problems, and have been linked to potential reproductive problems.

• **Perchloroethylene (Perc):** This is a solvent often used in dry cleaning products and some carpet cleaners and has been linked to potential cancer risks. Always hang dry cleaning outside or in a ventilated garage to dry for at least 48 hours.

• **1,4-dioxane:** This is a byproduct of the manufacturing process for certain cleaning ingredients, and has been linked to potential cancer risks.

• **Nonylphenol ethoxylates (NPEs), AKA Nonylphenol ethoxylate surfactants, Nonoxynols, Alkylphenol ethoxylates, Nonylphenol polyethylene glycol ethers,**

Nonylphenol polyoxyethylene ethers, Nonionic surfactants: These are surfactants often used in cleaning products that have been linked to potential hormone disruption, including estrogenic effects.

- **Ammonium sulfate:** This is a common ingredient in household cleaning products that can cause skin irritation and respiratory problems and has been linked to potential developmental and reproductive effects.

- **Quaternium-15, AKA Dowicils and Azonium:** This is a preservative often used in cleaning products that can release formaldehyde and have been linked to potential cancer risks.

- **Diethanolamine (DEA):** This is a surfactant often used in cleaning products that can cause skin and eye irritation and has been linked to potential hormone disruption.

- **Phenols:** These are commonly used in disinfectants and have been linked to potential respiratory and skin irritation, as well as potential reproductive and developmental effects.

- **Methylene chloride:** This is a solvent often used in paint and varnish removers that can cause skin and eye irritation and has been linked to potential cancer risks.

- **Petroleum distillates:** These are solvents often used in cleaning products such as degreasers or oven cleaners and have been linked to potential respiratory problems and skin irritation.

- **Butane:** This is a propellant often used in aerosol cleaners that can be harmful if inhaled and has been linked to potential neurological effects.

Knowledge is power, and if you read labels, you will be able to make informed choices about what you are exposing your body to. Remember, just do your best. You don't need to change everything all at once, but as you minimize your chemical exposures, you will see significant improvements in your health and decrease your disease risk. If you want more information and support in this process, the Wilde Vitality Detoxification Course has extensive resources for this subject.

CHAPTER 17
MINDSET - EMOTIONAL DETOX

Whenever you detox, more than just your body is altered. There is always an emotional response. If you are present with yourself in this manner, you will be able to create awareness, heal, and release toxic emotions and behaviors.

I have detoxified people for almost 20 years, and as the toxicants are mobilized, behaviors are altered, and habits are retrained, everyone has emotional reactions to the process. You may come up against triggers concerning how you have been interacting with food, yourself, your loved ones, and your body. Be present with your body. Be aware of how you feel. Pay attention to what you say to yourself.

SHIFT YOUR INTERNAL DIALOGUE TO LOVING SELF-TALK

How healthy is your relationship with yourself? I recognize that I have had a habit of saying hurtful, harmful things to myself that I wouldn't even say to someone I disliked! Would you say the things you say to yourself to someone you loved? Like a child? You very well may have heard those hurtful words as a child and internalized them into your own inner voice. Let's break the cycle of violence and neglect that you have aimed at yourself. Can you imagine how it would feel to show up as powerfully and lovingly for yourself as you would for a stray animal or marginalized population? What if you consciously released yourself from sabotage and shifted your dialogue and the feelings you have for yourself into those of self-love and self-care? Don't you think it is time to show up for yourself as you would others? To commit to supporting yourself? I do.

Try these actions and exercises to increase your self-love.

Take Action: The C word — Commit.

Look at yourself in the mirror, and commit to yourself. Do you vow to love and cherish yourself? For richer, for poorer, in sickness and in health? How can you commit to promising that to someone else if you haven't done it for yourself? Write down your vows or promises and post them somewhere you will see them often.

Take action: Look into your eyes every day and commit.

Say "*I do*" to you and living your best life.

Take action: Practice the emotion of self-love.

Do a little meditation every morning and embody love and appreciation for yourself. If negative thoughts surface, sit with them, recognize them, and use your mindset tools to let them go. What you pay attention to persists. Focus on gratitude and being happy and healthy, and it will become your reality. What you give your attention to grows.

This can be profoundly healing in more ways than one. I have regularly had clients go through a detox and then not fit into their lives anymore. They leave behind things that are unhealthy for them and become healthier, happier, and more fulfilled versions of themselves.

Take action: Write yourself positive affirmations and post them around your house.

This will help reprogram your mind for positivity. Write your favorite things about yourself. Make sure you believe them. Examples:

- I am fun!

- I am loving!

- I am a great mother, sister, friend, pet owner, employee, dancer, painter, driver, etc.!

Take action: Become aware.

Now, let's get a little vulnerable and honest. When you look in the mirror at yourself, what do you say that doesn't serve you? Be honest. We all do it. If I'm on autopilot, when I look in the mirror, I usually tell myself I'm getting old and fat. When I catch myself doing that outdated and unhealthy behavior, I say something else. I really look into my own eyes and shift. I say something sweet to myself, but it has to be something I believe. I'm not about to blow smoke up my own ass. I'm not into that. So, what do you say? What immediately comes to mind when you see your belly or ass, your gray hair, acne, or laugh lines in the mirror? Pay attention.

I have a soul sister named Anna Kate, and her mother, Barbara, raised her to be a self-confident and powerful woman in a generation of women who never feel as though they are good enough. One trick was to choose three parts of her body that were undoubtedly her best features. Anna Kate has the most beautiful feet – she knows it, and she will tell you. When she isn't feeling like a hot tamale in other areas of her life or in her physical looks, she can look down and appreciate her beautiful feet. What are your three body parts that are supermodel-worthy?

Take action: Change your story.

Words have the power to shift your reality, but if you don't believe something, it doesn't matter whether you read it daily or say it to yourself.

If you believe you are ugly and say that to yourself in the mirror every day, reading "*I am beautiful*" isn't going to shift that energy as effectively as something you do believe. I have "*I surrender*" written on my mirror in red lipstick. Initially, I wanted to write "*I give up*" until a dear friend recommended "*I surrender*" instead. Can you feel the difference?

There is a spectrum of emotional words, spanning from hopeless and "*no will to live*" to ecstatic joy and unconditional love.

You can use a stepwise process to ascend the spiral. Be sure to believe it. For example, you can move from "I am unworthy" to "I am despairing," which isn't as low on the feeling spectrum.

From "*I am despairing,*" you can move to "*I am a failure*" or "*I am angry.*"

From anger, you can admit that you are fearful or overwhelmed.

From being overwhelmed, you may be able to choose hopefulness.

From hope, you can choose to be curious. Curious about how to feel better or how to heal. This process can continue in a stepwise manner until you can regularly shift into powerful, positive emotions from those that initially appear negative.

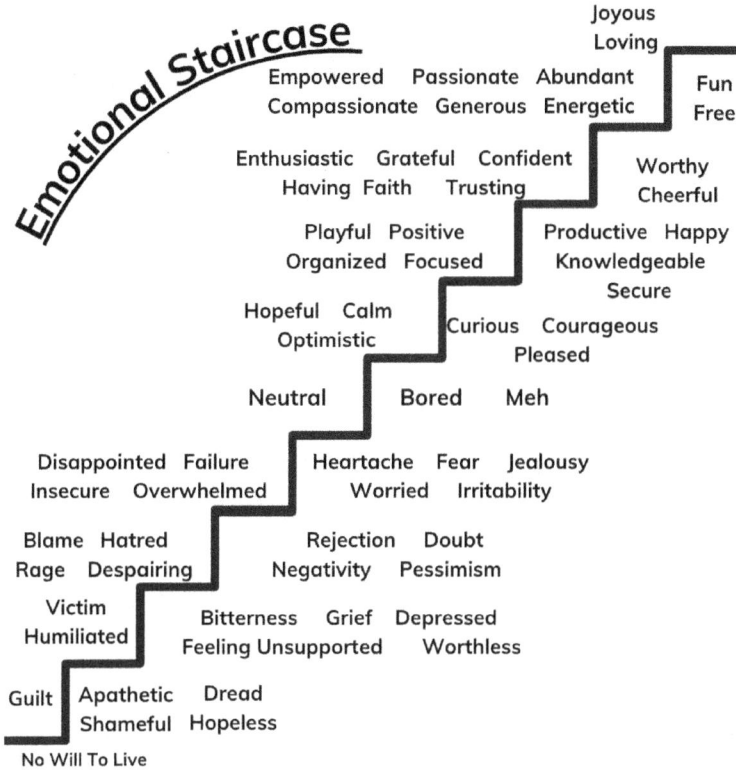

Emotional Staircase

Joyous
Loving

Empowered Passionate Abundant   Fun
Compassionate Generous Energetic   Free

Enthusiastic Grateful Confident   Worthy
Having Faith   Trusting   Cheerful

Playful Positive   Productive Happy
Organized Focused   Knowledgeable
                                        Secure

Hopeful Calm
Optimistic   Curious Courageous
                               Pleased

Neutral   Bored   Meh

Disappointed Failure   Heartache Fear Jealousy
Insecure   Overwhelmed   Worried Irritability

Blame Hatred   Rejection Doubt
Rage Despairing   Negativity Pessimism

Victim
Humiliated   Bitterness Grief Depressed
                  Feeling Unsupported   Worthless

Guilt Apathetic Dread
       Shameful Hopeless
No Will To Live

Fig 1: People feel different emotions differently and use different words to describe different emotions. This illustration is merely a guide to help you identify that some emotions feel better than others, and you can navigate up, or down, in a stepwise manner by identifying how you feel, and choosing a direction.

You can do the same with negative self-talk.

Instead of "*I am fat*".

Choose something more positive but believable.

I am strong.

I am healthy.

I am curvy.

I am sexy.

I am in the process of becoming my perfect size and shape.

You choose what you believe. Choose healthy, empowering thoughts. Words have power.

MEDITATION

How can you create a healthy, loving, and supportive relationship with your true self and what you conceive of as the great power of the universe? Meditation. I love the saying that if you don't have time to meditate for 20 minutes a day, you should meditate for 2 hours. I am one of those people. Meditation is beneficial for just about everything your body needs help with.

Healthy brains mean healthy, happy humans. Studies have shown that meditation is one of the best ways to protect your body from stress. While too much exercise can be harmful, there's no such thing as too much meditation! People regularly say they "can't meditate." Do you know what you can do? Breathe! Just breathe. Breathe in and out, and just do nothing for 3 minutes, then expand the time to 5 minutes and then to 20 minutes.

Detach from your "monkey mind"—the chatterbox that is your ego and internal dialogue, and all the limitations and poison it pours in your ear. Watch your thoughts; just watch them. Your brain will tell you all the things you need to do, could be doing, have done in the past, etc. It will perform mental gymnastics to get you to stop being present and get up and do something else.

So set a timer, commit to it, and don't get up until it goes off. There are tons of free apps and meditations on YouTube to guide you along your meditation journey. Find what you like. Insight Timer is a great place to start because it has a wide variety, many of which are short and tailored to what is currently troubling you. I often opt for the Tibetan bell option. I follow the sound and breathe, and when I think, "*Oh shit! I have to do X, Y, and Z or my life is going to fall apart in the next 30 seconds!*" I call 'bullshit', and I breathe some more and listen to the bells.

Recognize that your mind is both a fantastic tool and a terrible master. Breathe, and feel yourself in your body. You are driving the most magnificent bit of quantum machinery that exists in the known universe. Feel what that feels like. Breathe. Smile.

Take action: Choose supportive relationships.

You may experience loved ones giving their opinion about what you are doing with your health and life choices as you implement positive changes. Remember that their negative reactions to you choosing yourself and your health adventure to live your best life say way more about them than it does about you.

If they tell you:

- You are losing weight too fast.
- Your diet is unhealthy.
- Your diet is dangerous.
- Organic food doesn't matter.
- Detoxes don't work.

- The CDC and FDA can be trusted.

These statements aren't factual and are more of a reflection on them than on you. If you put rats in a bucket, none of them will escape. If one gets close to climbing out, the others will pull it back in.

You are part of your environment. When you change, you may experience others being triggered or uncomfortable by the changes you are committed to making for yourself and your health because they aren't willing to make them themselves. If people around you are not supportive of your health and choices, you can choose to expose yourself to their company and comments... or not. You have the power of choice.

Do you feel strong, supported, and happy around someone? Then keep hanging out with them! If you feel judged or negative around someone, that affords you an opportunity to choose whether you think they are healthy for you at this time... or not. Whether you want to detoxify your life from negative influences on your well-being... or not. Performance coaches tout that you are a combination of the five people you spend the most time with. Choose those people wisely.

On the other hand, this is one of the adages that I find true:

"If you want to change the world, start with yourself."
~Someone super annoying

As you shift into a stronger, more powerful, healthier, and more balanced place, the world changes around you. I used to drink heavily during family holidays and even had an emergency joint for when things got completely out of hand. I was enraged by people around me as they triggered my childhood wounds and patterns. I wanted nothing to do with any of them for years and only sporadically spent time with them out of obligation.

But things got better with time. I promise you, when you show up differently, the world around you changes. Please don't misunderstand me; I have created magnificent boundaries and clear expectations about how I deserve to be treated. I don't associate with negative, dishonest, unkind, or abusive people; I don't care who they are or who they are related to. You don't deserve to be exposed to poor relationships either, and you too can choose how you are treated.

My relationships with all the members of my family are much more positive, fulfilling, and loving than they were two years ago. It has nothing to do with them. I took responsibility for my reactions, worked with my inner child and the wounds that I created, and practiced radical and honest forgiveness.

"If you think you are enlightened, go and spend a week with your family."
~Ram Dass

I'm not enlightened, but I do have a much better relationship with them, even though a full week is honestly pushing it. Much of their behavior hasn't changed, but some of it has.

At one point during an especially excruciating part of my wellness journey process, I yelled, *"How can I ever forgive them?! For what they did to me?!"*

I am not a victim, and I recognize that I played my part in our estrangement and dysfunction. If I can't forgive them when they are the ones who wiped my ass as a baby and fed and sheltered me for the first 20 years of my life, who can I forgive? If I can't forgive my blood or my family, what does that say about the kind of person I am?

"Not forgiving someone is like drinking poison every day and hoping they die."
~Malachy McCourt

Choose how you deserve to be treated. Find your tribe and the people who fill you up with love and laughter. Create healthy boundaries, and then let the past go. Forgive others, and more importantly, forgive yourself. Allow for the fact that people can change. Everyone is just one choice away from being a more loving member of our society, and let's allow the space for them to choose that adventure.

Until then, you don't have to share yourself, your time, or your energy with them. You may be surprised; however, as you work on yourself, others are inspired to change as well. No one lives in a vacuum, and small butterfly-wing changes can create transformational storms.

LIVE WITH INTENTION

Are you a lion? Do you want to create your best life with power and vitality? Or a sheep? Do you want to live a life of quiet desperation, getting offended about things that don't impact your life at all, and staying with the flock of mediocrity? If you are a lion, create a map to help guide you along your journey.

Take a couple of moments every morning and set a few intentions that will get you closer to your primary health and life goals. Setting intentions can have a powerful impact on success, both in your personal and professional lives.

Starting the day with clear and focused goals sets the tone for a productive and successful day ahead. By taking the time to reflect on what you wish to achieve and setting intentions, you can align your thoughts, emotions, and actions toward your desired outcomes. This helps to increase focus, motivation, and a sense of purpose, which are essential ingredients for success. Setting intentions can help energetically and emotionally and also support the prioritization of your tasks and responsibilities for the day.

By having a clear understanding of what you want to achieve and the importance it has, you are better equipped to make decisions, allocate time and resources effectively, and stay on track toward your goals. Be sure to prioritize your intentions for self-care and rest. It may seem counterintuitive, but this leads to increased productivity, improved time management, and reduced stress levels.

Commit to excellence and ensure success by completing at least one of these processes every day. Make time for them and yourself. What are you doing for self-care? Treat yourself to a massage, a nap, or even a mini-spa day at home full of luxurious rest and self-care. These quiet, contemplative times are important to allow your body to work optimally, get into the parasympathetic system of rest, digest, and repair, and optimize your body's ability to detoxify. Take the time for yourself, make yourself a priority, and enjoy reflecting on the new life you are creating with power and vision.

Most of us need to shift our daily rituals toward those that serve us rather than those that just help us survive. Mindfully creating intentions to work toward goals can help instill new habits for you to become the best version of yourself in your life. Set intentions, list out your self-care tasks for the day, and create healthy habits to ensure your success.

Research in the field of neuroscience has shown that the brain is wired to seek out rewards and reinforce positive behaviors. When you complete a task, your brain releases dopamine, the neurotransmitter associated with feelings of pleasure, reward, and satisfaction. This release of dopamine reinforces the behavior and creates a desire to repeat it in the future, making it easier to form new habits. The repeated formation of new habits leads to the creation of neural pathways in the brain, which are the foundation for new patterns of behavior. So, check off things on your list, give yourself a high five, and enjoy that dopamine dump, baby!

You probably intuitively know that creating positive habits is a crucial factor in success. When you program yourself with supportive behaviors, they operate unconsciously and free up cognitive resources, allowing you to focus your attention on your next goals and the important tasks needed to achieve them.

I designed The Wilde Life Planner to guide you in the creation of healthy habits, so take a moment and imagine how powerful creating a new default operating system will be, feel how your body will feel as it becomes healthier, and see what a difference it will make in your life. Then, commit to creating a habit of using it!

CHAPTER 18
DIGITAL DETOX

The internet is, IMO, both the best and worst invention in recent history. We can hold supercomputers in our hands and access almost limitless information at all times. On the other side, we are exposed to highly addictive, dopamine-hit-inducing screens. Our digital diet is part of our "consumption," and it offers constant advertising for meaningless materialism, hormone-disrupting blue light, social starvation in a sea of plenty, and cultural sicknesses we haven't even begun to understand.

We do know that the more time a child spends on a screen, the less able they are to imagine. Let that sink in. Screens are killing imagination. Imagination has played a critical role in human consciousness and culture throughout history. It is through imagination that we have been able to create and express our deepest desires, fears, and beliefs, giving birth to art, literature, music, and other forms of creative expression.

Imagination has also played a vital role in shaping our cultural identity by allowing us to explore different worldviews and perspectives and to communicate complex ideas in a way that transcends language and cultural barriers. Ultimately, imagination has been a driving force behind human progress and innovation, and it continues to shape our world and our understanding of ourselves and others. We are crippling our children and the next generation by preventing them from exercising their imaginations because it is easier to put them in front of a screen than to engage them, entertain them, and give them attention. I think this is one of the real causes of attention deficit disorders; parents are so overwhelmed from every direction that the screens help them manage their lives by keeping their kids safe and quiet. But this not only steals the imagination from children; research has shown that screen exposure and digital media can have an addictive nature similar to that of drugs or other substances.

One of the reasons for this addiction is the effect that screens have on our neurotransmitter metabolism. Neurotransmitters are chemicals in the brain that transmit signals between neurons, and they play a crucial role in regulating our mood, behavior, and cognitive function. Digital media exposure, particularly social media, has been shown to trigger the release of dopamine, a neurotransmitter associated with pleasure and reward. The release of dopamine creates a sense of pleasure and reinforces our desire to engage in these activities repeatedly, leading to addiction.

To add insult to injury, prolonged exposure to screens can cause changes in the structure and function of our brain, affecting our cognitive and emotional development. Studies have shown that excessive screen time can lead to decreased gray matter in areas of the brain responsible for processing information, decision-making, attention, and impulse control, leading to impulsive behavior and difficulty focusing.

The impact on cognitive function can also lead to a decreased ability to empathize with others, becoming desensitized to the emotional experiences of others, and having lower levels of memory, attention, and language skills. Does this explain the asinine behavior of your ex-husband or ex-wife too? Screen exposure has also been linked to behavioral problems in children, including attention deficit hyperactivity disorder (ADHD) and aggression. Research has shown that children who spend more time in front of screens have higher rates of ADHD symptoms, and excessive screen use has been associated with increased levels of aggression and impulsivity.

There is a growing concern about the negative impacts of digital dependency on our health and well-being. Digital detoxification is a way to reduce our dependence on these devices and regain control over our lives.

First and foremost, excessive use of digital devices can lead to a sedentary lifestyle, which is associated with various health problems such as obesity, heart disease, and diabetes. People who spend long hours in front of their screens are less likely to engage in physical activity, which is essential for maintaining a healthy body and mind. Digital detoxification can help you break this cycle of sedentary behavior and encourage you to be more active.

Moreover, excessive use of digital devices can hurt your mental health. Studies have shown that social media use is associated with increased rates of anxiety, depression, and other mental health issues. Social media platforms can create a sense of FOMO (fear of missing out) and trigger feelings of inadequacy and low self-esteem. Digital detoxification can help you break free from the comparison trap and focus on what truly matters in your life.

Another reason why digital detoxification is important is that it can help you improve your relationships with others. Digital devices have transformed the way we communicate with each other, but they have also made us less present in the moment. You have probably become accustomed to checking your phone and responding to messages even when you are in the company of others. Digital detoxification helps you in being more mindful and present in your interactions with others, which can improve your relationships and overall happiness.

Furthermore, detoxing from digital devices can help improve your sleep quality. The blue light emitted by digital devices disrupts your circadian rhythm and makes it harder for you to fall asleep at night. Studies have shown that people who use their phones before bedtime have poorer sleep quality and are more likely to experience insomnia. By reducing your screen time before bedtime, you improve your sleep quality and wake up feeling more rested and energized.

By reducing your dependence on digital devices, you can improve your physical health, mental health, relationships with others, and sleep quality. It may be challenging to disconnect from your devices because they are designed to be addictive! Commit to taking breaks from the constant stimulation and allowing yourself to recharge and reconnect with the world around you. Take the time to unplug and enjoy the simple pleasures of life that you often overlook when you are zoned out and consuming meaningless ephemera in the digital world. Look at your screen time tracker on your phone, log how much time you spend mindlessly scrolling through something that doesn't exist, and choose to do something with your hands and body other than swipe, like, comment, share, follow, binge watch, or repost.

I challenge you to spend your free time doing something that doesn't include a screen or digital device for a full week.

TAKE ACTION

- Play cards or a board game
- Cook a new recipe
- Read a "real" book
- Go for a walk, run, hike, or bike
- Connect with a pet
- Play with a child
- Do yoga
- Do a puzzle or crossword
- Paint or sculpt
- Crochet, sew, or knit
- Build something
- Garden
- Daydream

HOBBIES

Imagine yourself in a world where the hustle and bustle of everyday life has taken over. From the moment you wake up to the moment you go to bed, you are constantly bombarded with to-do lists, deadlines, emails, notifications, and responsibilities. Oh, wait... You are likely living in this world right now, and it can be challenging to take a step back and focus on yourself.

Amidst the demands of work, social obligations, and family responsibilities, we often neglect to indulge in activities that bring us joy and relaxation. This is where hobbies come in: they offer a respite from the stresses of life and can have a profound impact on our health and well-being. Research has shown that engaging in hobbies can bring numerous benefits, both physical and mental. One of the most evident advantages is stress relief. Hobbies provide an escape from the daily grind, allowing you to focus on something you enjoy and take your mind off of your worries. This can lead to decreased levels of cortisol, the hormone responsible for stress, and a subsequent improvement in mood.

In addition to reducing stress, hobbies can also enhance cognitive function. Whether it's painting, playing an instrument, or solving puzzles, engaging in activities that require focus and mental effort can help keep the brain sharp and improve memory. Studies have shown that older adults who engage in hobbies have a lower risk of cognitive decline and dementia.

Hobbies can have physical benefits as well. Participating in activities such as gardening, hiking, or dancing can increase physical activity levels and improve cardiovascular health. Additionally, hobbies that require fine motor skills, such as knitting or woodworking, can improve hand-eye coordination and dexterity.

Perhaps one of the most significant benefits of hobbies is the sense of fulfillment they provide. In a world where you may often feel like you're just going through the motions, hobbies offer a sense of purpose and accomplishment. Whether it's completing a challenging puzzle or finishing a painting, hobbies give you something tangible to show for your efforts and can boost self-esteem, self-worth, and confidence. Of course, not all hobbies are equal when it comes to health benefits. While watching TV or scrolling through social media may be enjoyable, they don't provide the same level of cognitive or physical stimulation as other activities. Think of them as junk food rather than a green smoothie for your brain. It's essential to choose hobbies that challenge and engage you to reap the full benefits.

So, what makes a good hobby? It depends. What works for one person may not work for another. However, some key factors to consider when choosing a hobby include enjoyment, challenge, and fulfillment. If you dread the thought of engaging in a particular activity, it's unlikely to provide the stress relief and sense of fulfillment that hobbies are meant to offer. Even if it is exercise. Am I right? You will not see me in a Zumba class, but give me a chance to walk in the mountains for 15 miles, and I will take it. Hobbies should be challenging enough to provide a sense of accomplishment, but not so difficult that they become frustrating or suck the fun out of life. We get enough of that already.

It is crucial to make time for hobbies in your busy life. It's all too easy to prioritize pressing obligations over the things you enjoy—the behaviors that feed your mind, build your body, and lift your spirit. Prioritizing hobbies is prioritizing an aspect of your self-care and can increase the likelihood of negative consequences for your health and well-being. Whether it's carving out a few hours on the weekends or making time before or after work, like everything else, finding a regular time to engage in hobbies can help make them a consistent and beneficial part of your life.

So, what are some hobbies that can provide these fantastic benefits? There are countless options out there, but here are a few examples:

Artistic pursuits: Painting, drawing, sculpting,

or even coloring books can provide an excellent creative outlet and improve your mood. Physical activities: Running, hiking, swimming, or playing sports can improve your cardiovascular health and overall physical fitness.

Crafting: Knitting, crocheting, or sewing can improve dexterity and provide a sense of accomplishment. If you like putting models together, don't sniff too much airplane glue and be sure to wear a respirator.

Reading and writing: Reading can be a fantastic escape from reality, and writing can provide a creative outlet.

Gardening: Planting and tending a garden can provide a sense of relaxation and accomplishment, as well as improve your grip strength and overall physical fitness. Research has shown that getting your hands dirty in the garden increases levels of serotonin in the brain.

But what if you're not sure what you enjoy doing? Or are you bored with the old things that used to amuse you? That's okay, too! Spice it up by exploring new hobbies. Life can be a wonderful adventure of exploration and learning. If you continue to expand into new areas of interest, you will not only keep yourself busy and entertained, but you could end up being the most interesting person in a room.

Here are a few tips for finding new hobbies:

Try something new: Don't be afraid to try something you've never done before, whether it's a painting class or a dance lesson.

Ask for recommendations: Reach out to friends or family members who have hobbies they enjoy and ask for suggestions or to accompany them.

Explore your interests: Think about the things you enjoy and try to find a hobby that aligns with those interests.

"Is life not a thousand times too short for us to bore ourselves?"
~Friedrich Nietzsche

THE IMPORTANCE OF SELF-CARE

Self-care is the new Prada. I know people who have spent over $20,000 to improve their sleep. They recognized how important sleep was for their lives, committed to making it a priority, and allocated the necessary resources to make better sleep a priority. I'm sure you have seen the memes about *"If you say you don't have time for (insert whatever here), then it just isn't a priority."* #truth

In a world where "hustle culture" and "grind culture" seem to reign supreme, the importance of self-care often takes a backseat. We're constantly told to work harder, faster, and longer, all in the name of success and being able to brag on social media.

Research has shown that practicing self-care, such as regular exercise, healthy eating, and stress-reducing activities, can have profound effects on both your physical and mental health. No Way! I hope you were sitting down for that. Let's not forget the impact that self-care can have on your productivity and creativity. It's hard to be your best self when you're burned out and exhausted. But self-care isn't just about the occasional spa day or bubble bath. It's about recognizing that your own needs and desires are just as important as anyone else's. It's about setting healthy boundaries, advocating for yourself, and prioritizing your well-being.

Now, I know what you might be thinking: *"I don't have time for self-care!"* But here's the thing: Making time for self-care is a smart move. It means being intentional with your time and energy and recognizing that taking care of yourself is not a waste of time but an investment in yourself and your future.

And let's not forget that self-care looks different for everyone. It could be as simple as taking three deep breaths when you feel stressed and taking a walk outside during your lunch break, or as involved as seeking Jungian therapy or making time for an hour-long daily meditation practice. The key is to find what works for you and commit to making it a regular part of your routine. Then you can add it to your self-care routines when you start to see how it benefits every area of your life.

So, to all the hustlers and grinders out there, I challenge you to prioritize self-care. Take a break, go for a walk, or indulge in your favorite hobby. Set healthy boundaries, advocate for yourself, and recognize that your well-being is just as important as your success.

You spend your time, money, and energy on what you deem important. Sometimes those priorities are a bit screwy; for example, watching 8 hours of football on a Saturday, a Sunday, or both but saying there isn't time to get to the gym, call your mother, clean your bathroom, or do your taxes.

When you care for yourself with hobbies and health regimens, you fill your own cup so that you can give to others or more fully engage with your work or social priorities. Practicing self-care is not just a luxury; it's a savvy move. It's about investing in yourself and your future and recognizing that taking care of yourself is essential to achieving success. So go ahead, take a break, and take care of yourself; your success depends on it.

SELF-CARE IN THE CHAOS OF CHILDREARING

Parenting is the most difficult, undervalued, frightening, soul-crushing, and even frustrating activity a human can experience. Children are beautiful opportunities for us to face our "stuff" with grace and love, or anger and sorrow.

My son has had more access to screens than I ever thought he would. At first, it just started while we took plane trips. Then he got more iPad and TV time because I was so overwhelmed with the massive changes in my life that I dove into screen time with my kindle unlimited to numb my pain. At that time in my life, I was only capable of the bare minimum of self-care, and he and I both suffered from it.

Then, COVID. *Ugh.* After I dug myself out of my screen and other addictions and fully interacted with life in a meaningful way, we addressed his addiction and behaviors. It isn't easier or quieter than just plugging him into a screen, but it is so worth it. The only screens he now gets at my house are short periods he earns via chores and behavioral incentives, and family movie time. I am more engaged in his childhood and enjoy his company more now that we choose to have less screen exposure. But we had to create boundaries and expectations so I have time for me, as well as time for him.

Remember, your children are always watching.

Children Learn What They Live

If children live with criticism, they learn to condemn.
If children live with hostility, they learn to fight.
If children live with ridicule, they learn to be shy.
If children live with shame, they learn to feel guilty.
If children live with encouragement, they learn confidence.
If children live with tolerance, they learn to be patient.
If children live with praise, they learn to appreciate.
If children live with acceptance, they learn to love.
If children live with approval, they learn to like themselves.
If children live with honesty, they learn truthfulness.
If children live with security, they learn to have faith in themselves and others.
If children live with friendliness, they learn the world is a nice place in which to live.

~Dorothy Law Nolte

As digital devices become increasingly ubiquitous, it is essential to teach your children to use them in a responsible and balanced way. By restricting screen time, children can develop important life skills, such as creativity, problem-solving, and critical thinking, that are essential for success in the 21st century. By prioritizing activities such as exercise, reading, and spending time outdoors, children can build resilience, self-discipline, self-care regimens, and social skills that will serve them well throughout their lives.

Limiting screen time can help foster a deeper connection between children and the world around them. By engaging in activities that encourage exploration and discovery, children can develop a sense of curiosity and wonder that will inspire them to pursue their passions and make meaningful contributions to society.

It isn't just about a deeper connection to their friends and the rest of the world, but also with you, their parent or caretaker, and the rest of the family and social circle. The quality of parent-child interactions has a profound impact on children's health and success. Positive parent-child relationships have been linked to better physical health, emotional well-being, and academic achievement through responsive and nurturing interactions.

Conscious caretakers, mindfully creating time for connection, provide children with a sense of security and emotional support, which are essential for healthy development. These interactions can help children build self-esteem, develop resilience, and learn important social skills that will serve them well throughout their lives.

Parents and caretakers who prioritize spending quality time with their children invest in academic success and achievement over the long term. By providing support and encouragement, parents can help children develop a love of learning and a sense of curiosity that will inspire them to pursue their goals and aspirations, as well as the self-esteem necessary to believe that they too can live their best life and see their dreams come true. As you model self-care, you can help promote healthy habits and behaviors in the children and adolescents you interact with. When you exercise, eat well, enjoy good sleep habits, enforce healthy boundaries, and foster loving relationships, children are watching and learning how to develop lifelong habits that will promote their health and well-being. They may scream and cry and act out like crack addicts when you first take away the screens, but I promise, you will see your child raise their eyes from a make-believe world designed to addict them and make them mindless consumers of plastic shit and social drivel. You will see them engage in life in new and meaningful ways where their personalities and intelligence will shine, so they too can sing the song they came here to sing. And that is priceless.

CHAPTER 19
DAILY DETOX BOOSTS

Isn't it a brilliantly empowering notion—the idea of actively bolstering your body's natural detoxification processes, regardless of whether you're in the midst of a detox regimen or not? I'm inclined to agree wholeheartedly. That's why, in this chapter, we're delving into the art of seamlessly integrating detox-enhancing practices into your daily life.

Picture this: a life where every choice you make contributes to your well-being, guiding you steadily toward a state of optimal health. I'm thrilled to introduce you to my collection of Wilde Life Health Hacks. These are the little shifts that can make a monumental difference.

EMBARKING ON YOUR DETOX JOURNEY - EVERY SINGLE DAY

Detoxification isn't a one-time event; it's an ongoing symphony of self-care that your body performs ceaselessly. By weaving detox-boosting behaviors into the habits of your life, you're offering your body a foundation of support—a chorus of nourishment that reverberates with vitality. Imagine the power of daily habits that shield you from the onslaught of toxicants, ensuring your body's channels of elimination remain clear and unencumbered. These simple yet potent habits can radiate positive effects far beyond detoxification, illuminating your path toward a life of vigor and longevity.

EMBRACE YOUR INNER WILDE: UNVEILING HEALTH HACKS

I'm excited to share with you a curated selection of Wilde Life Health Hacks—strategies that have been refined and polished over years of experience. These aren't mere temporary fixes; they're your new default programming—habits that effortlessly integrate into your routine, gradually enhancing your well-being.

From the moment you wake to the time you lay your head to rest, these hacks will be your constant companions, working synergistically to invigorate your body and mind.

So, are you ready to step into a life where each day is a journey that creates health and vitality? Are you eager to seize the opportunity to fuel your body's innate detox powers and revel in the radiance it brings? Get ready to transform your life from the ground up, one health hack at a time.

In the pages ahead, we'll explore these Wilde Life Health Hacks in detail, unraveling their benefits and revealing how seamlessly they can be integrated into your existence. You can join my 30-day Healthy Morning Routine Challenge via my YouTube channel, Facebook, or Instagram. Prepare to embrace the art of daily detoxification-boosting behaviors and let your vitality flourish like never before. The journey starts now! As an Amazon Associate, I earn money from qualifying purchases.

DRINK PLENTY OF PURIFIED, STRUCTURED WATER

A simple guideline is to drink half your body weight in ounces of purified, structured water a day. That means if you weigh 200 lbs., 100 oz of water a day is an excellent place to start getting you hydrated. I drink my weight in ounces because the more hydrated you are, the better your body works. We cannot overemphasize the importance of filtering your water sources to ensure you get clean water and do not add to your toxic load. Remember, for every caffeinated or alcoholic drink you have, you need to drink just as much water to balance it out. If you are up urinating a lot at night, you can stop drinking a couple of hours before bed. If that doesn't resolve it, drink most of your water earlier in the day. You want clean, filtered water, and be sure to drink it out of glass or stainless steel. I love these water bottle options.

- Stainless steel

- Glass

My favorite filtration system is the Berkey, a stainless-steel gravity-fed countertop water dispenser. You have several sizes to choose from, depending on your family's needs. I have a larger size because I don't just use it for drinking water. I also use it for cooking and filtering the water I give my pets and plants. Whatever model you choose, make sure you get both black and white filters for the best filtration. Other family members have the smaller capacity Berkey's, and it just can't keep up with the water use of one person, let alone several.

I'm not a fan of reverse osmosis (RO) water because the process wastes a lot of water and uses a ton of electricity, along with the fact that the RO water needs to have minerals added back in so you can absorb it optimally. Without re-mineralizing, it can leach minerals out of your body, which is one of the last things you want to do. If you want to remineralize and add electrolytes to your water with flavor, I love the Electrolyte Supreme by Jigsaw Health, and they come in several flavors.

WHAT IS STRUCTURED WATER?

Ideally, you can fill up your glass or stainless-steel water bottle with your Berkey filter of choice and make "structured water." Structured water is a charged form of water molecules that occur when water falls from the sky, runs over rocks in waterfalls, flows in rivers, and succumbs to the tides of lakes. Isn't that poetic? It is the form of water found in nature, and surprise, surprise, it is the best kind for us.

When you run water through a filter or water treatment plant, it loses this natural charge. Structured water is crucial because it makes your cells more able to absorb and use the water you drink. Dr. Gerald Pollack is a bioengineer and researcher who has studied the properties of water and its potential health benefits. According to Dr. Pollack, structured water may have several benefits for human health, including improved hydration, increased energy levels, and reduced oxidative stress.

You don't need to buy a fancy machine to make it. You can simply stir a mason jar full of water in a clockwise direction and put it in the refrigerator.

I recommend reading the book *The Hidden Messages in Water* by Masaru Emoto. You may be inspired to write messages on your water containers to imbue them with intentions like "love", "health", "happiness", "joy", etc. You certainly may avoid "Liquid Death". Whether you subscribe to the power of intentions and energy or not, simply being mindful of what you put in your body is powerful in and of itself. When you think of your body with love, everything improves.

Choose water from clean sources that is, ideally, bottled in glass. If you must drink from a plastic bottle, get a more substantial one rather than the really thin options. The thinner the plastic, the more likely it is to put nasty phthalates, BPA, and other toxicants into the water if it heats up. Never keep filled plastic water bottles in a place where they can get hot, no matter if they are made from hard plastic. Regardless of the hardness of the plastic, it is releasing microplastics into your foods and beverages. #fuckplastic

EAT WILDE

Be conscious of what you consume and choose food that actually counts as "food", rather than a chemically based food product specifically designed to alter your body and brain chemistry so you want to eat more. And more. And more. Even though it doesn't really provide anything other than neuroactive chemicals and sugar.

Choose organic food to help decrease the number of pesticides you are exposed to in your diet and reduce the burden on your body to detoxify. While organic foods aren't perfectly clean, they have less toxicity than conventionally grown crops. People often complain about the cost of organic food, but disease is much more expensive than a couple of extra dollars spent on higher-quality groceries.

Eating a spectrum of colorful vegetables and low-glycemic fruits is one of the most important things you can do to help detoxify your body and decrease disease because they provide a great dietary source of essential fiber, nutrients, antioxidants, bioflavonoids, vitamins, and minerals. Low-glycemic fruits don't spike your blood sugar and support increased lipolysis and weight loss.

High-quality protein helps your entire body function better, aids weight loss, and repairs physical body damage, while EPA and DHA support the strength of every cell in your body along with healthy inflammation and optimized brain health.

Allow yourself some treats and some comfort food - some times. But pay attention to how you feel after you eat it. You may find that the short-term taste sensation isn't worth the long-term consequences.

SWEAT AND SUPPORT YOUR SKIN!

One of the more concerning things that I hear from patients is that they don't sweat. Screw the old idea that "men and horses sweat, women only glow." If you have any health issues that can be caused by toxicity—hello, most are! Then you need to incorporate sweating into your daily life.

Stay away from antiperspirants that stop you from sweating, too. If you read the back of every antiperspirant container, it will caution you to "consult your doctor before using if you have kidney disease." Something in antiperspirant (aluminum) is so potentially toxic to the human body (linked to dementia) that you are in trouble if your kidneys can't clear it out well. Kidney function progressively decreases after the age of 40, and a lot of adults have kidney disease. So, switch to deodorants and allow yourself to sweat!

Repeated sauna usage helps restore the skin's toxin elimination ability. This is possibly the most effective way to train yourself to sweat. Released toxins from deep inside the body are eliminated from the body by sweat and/or through the intestinal tract. You can use this link to order an excellent home sauna that is medical-grade and portable. If you have a little more money and space, I recommend a wooden one with a sound system, an air purifier, and color therapy.

DRY SKIN BRUSHING

Lymph is an extracellular fluid found in between the cells and performs a vital function for the body. It is the fluid caught in your tissues when you have swelling or edema, and it provides a means for cells to get rid of waste from their normal metabolism.

The lymphatic system is a network of vessels and tissues that helps filter waste and toxins from the body. It is believed that dry skin brushing can help stimulate the lymphatic system and improve its ability to remove waste and toxins from the body. By promoting lymphatic drainage, dry skin brushing may also help to reduce swelling and improve the overall health and appearance of the skin.

Your lymph system has lymph nodes that house some of your immune system cells and functions overall to help fluid from your cells return to the cardiovascular system after being cleaned and filtered. It is not directly connected to the heart, arteries, or veins and depends upon muscle contractions to return the lymph fluid to circulation, where toxicants are excreted by the liver and kidneys. So, again, MYA.

Dry skin brushing is a technique in which a brush with firm bristles is used to massage the skin in a specific pattern. It should always be done in the direction of your heart, especially if you are prone to edema and swelling. The idea is to brush your skin lightly to remove dead cells and exfoliate, but it also brings circulation to your tissue to help clean it out. This is a great kit to help move the lymph in the body back into circulation, where it can be filtered. It is said to improve circulation, remove dead skin cells, promote lymphatic drainage, and even help reduce cellulite!

MYA (MOVE YOUR ASS)

Movement is good for just about everything. Don't forget that MYA also plays a key role in detoxification by increasing circulation, balancing hormones, helping your digestive system work optimally, and sweating out toxins!

POOP!

Constipation is extremely unhealthy and a root cause of many health issues. One of the worst things you can do during detox is not eliminate your bowels at least once a day. If you are chronically constipated, you are more likely to have an autoimmune disease, allergies, hormone imbalances, colon cancer, and metabolic issues. More and more research is coming out showing the importance of a healthy microbiome, or the probiotics in your gut. A balanced microbiome can help with bowel regularity and digestive health, support your immune system, mental health, metabolism, cardiovascular health, and even decrease inflammation. If you have trouble with your elimination (pooping), check out our resources to help you. I developed this Leaky Gut Power Powder, and I recommend it to everyone having digestive issues. I had a client buy 10 bags as gifts for their family and loved ones this past holiday season. It works.

EMBODY YOUR BITCH BE COOL!

Emotional stress short-circuits the processes in your body that help you detoxify and repair. It increases your sympathetic (fight, flight, and freeze) system and decreases your parasympathetic (rest, digest, and repair) system. Commit to managing your stress in beneficial and healthy ways. Not booze, eating emotionally, or other addictions.

- **Exercise:** Regular physical activity can help reduce stress and improve mood by releasing endorphins, the body's natural feel-good chemicals.

- **Breathing exercises:** Slow, deep breathing can help calm the mind and reduce feelings of stress and anxiety.

- **Mindfulness meditation**: This involves focusing on the present moment and allowing thoughts and feelings to pass by without judgment. It has been shown to reduce stress and improve mental well-being. Being fully present with your experience at the moment eradicates depression and anxiety. Anxiety can only exist in the future; depression can exist in the past.

- **Nature walks:** Spending time in nature has been shown to reduce stress and improve mood.

- **Social support:** Spending time with friends and family or participating in social activities can provide emotional support and help reduce stress.

- **Yoga:** This practice combines physical postures with deep breathing and mindfulness and has been shown to reduce stress and improve mental well-being.

- **Progressive muscle relaxation:** This

technique involves tensing and relaxing different muscle groups and has been shown to reduce muscle tension and stress.

- **Neuro-Linguistic Programming:** This type of therapy helps individuals identify and change negative thought patterns and behaviors that contribute to stress. It is the most revolutionary therapy I have found because it helps you completely rewire yourself for success. We all know what we SHOULD be doing, so why don't we? NLP empowers you to really change. You can book a full or mini-breakthrough with me, on my website.

- **Music therapy:** Listening to music, singing, or playing an instrument has been shown to reduce stress and improve mood.

- **Sleep:** Getting enough sleep is important for overall health and well-being and has been shown to reduce stress and improve mood.

STOP THE CHEMISTRY EXPERIMENT INSANITY

While you are working hard to detoxify or just swimming in the normal toxic soup of daily exposure, the last thing you want to do is add more toxicants to your system or slow down your body's ability to do its job.

The following is a list of factors that make detoxification more difficult:

- **Dehydration**

- **Constipation**

- **A pro-inflammatory diet:** one low in fiber, high in refined sugars, flours, saturated or trans-fats, artificial colors, artificial flavors, artificial sweeteners, preservatives, and alcohol. Eating up foods to which you are intolerant and sensitive is also pro-inflammatory; therefore, avoiding them is key. If you don't know which foods you are most sensitive to, you can get a food sensitivity panel on my website NaturopathicMD.com.

- **Over-the-counter and illegal drugs:** include cannabis, alcohol, caffeine, and nicotine.

- **Adding more chemicals:** like perfumes, air fresheners, plastics, etc.

So stop it. Choose your health adventure, and choose which toxicants you are most willing to be exposed to with full awareness that you will need to detoxify regularly to get them out. When I first started researching the health impacts of pollution in 2000, I was a bit freaked out because I saw the massive exposures and how little we could do about them. My diet consisted mostly of coffee, chocolate, champagne, and cigarettes because I reasoned that if I was going to be poisoned by pollution and GMOs, I might as well enjoy it.

These days, I knowingly make choices where I am exposed to toxicity because... I like them. For example, I choose to get my hair dyed regularly because I'm not ready to go gracefully gray. I used to use henna and indigo, natural herbs with zero toxins, but they no longer work for me due to the overwhelming number of gray hairs I have gotten over the past few years. I get my hair done, but I choose Aveda salons because they are supposed to be less toxic. I also take supplements designed to support liver function, glutathione production, and detox.

One of my other toxic sins to confess is that I love to get manicures and pedicures. I pretend I'm an

Egyptian queen getting my hands and feet rubbed with sacred oils. I've explored "vegan" nail colors and low-VOC nail polish to do at home, but I prefer the salon. So, I drink extra water the day I get my nails done and take my supplements to protect myself from the increased toxicity.

I eat seabass once a year, usually on my birthday. I never eat tuna or other high-mercury fish, no matter if they are my favorites. I eat fish and seafood mindfully and take precautions when I do so to decrease the absorption of the metals into my body.

Detoxifying regularly is part of my self-care regimen to decrease the long-term impacts of not only these toxic behaviors I choose to engage in but also the daily toxicants I am exposed to by simply living on this planet. It is easy to get overwhelmed by it all, and so it is important to have some fun while you are at it. That is why I named my podcast *The Bad Girls' Guide to Living Well*.

"You are allowed three vices in your life; and sex and chocolate don't count."
~Dr. Jim Sensenig

EFFECTIVELY FILTER YOUR AIR

I also avoid chemical exposure by filtering my air and water. My son has slept in a bedroom with an Austin Air filter since he was born. We have one in every bedroom and another for the bulk of the house. There is another in my office where I see patients because, while I have no control over forest fires and toxic emissions, I can control the indoor air I breathe.

Indoor air quality can also be improved by incorporating certain plants into the environment.

Having plants in your house is healthy! Who knew?

The following plants are commonly available and are known to remove pollutants and toxins like VOCs from the air, making it healthier to breathe.

- Spider plant (*Chlorophytum comosum)*
- Peace lily (*Spathiphyllum spp.)*
- Snake plant (*Sansevieria trifasciata*)
- Golden pathos (*Epipremnum aureum*)
- Rubber plant (*Ficus elastica*)
- Aloe vera (*Aloe barbadensis*)
- English ivy (*Hedera helix*)

Bringing nature into your home environment will help improve air quality and promote better health in various ways, but it does not replace adequate ventilation or minimizing exposure.

UNPLUG WITH A DIGITAL DETOX

"Kill Your Television" is my favorite bumper sticker. When you watch TV, you go into a suggestible, semi-hypnotic state where your brain can be programmed with commercials, infected with fear, and controlled by cultural pressures.

Taking a break from digital devices, lackluster TV, and social media can provide significant health benefits. It's like giving your brain a spa day—a chance to relax and rejuvenate without all the constant noise and stimulation. Research has shown that excessive screen time can lead to physical and mental health issues such as eye strain, disrupted sleep patterns, and a serious case of "meh-itis," in addition to the negative effects of EMF exposure we already discussed. But fear not, my digitally-addicted friends; a digital detox can help alleviate these issues and improve overall well-being.

Reducing screen time can help you become less like an insecure hermit crab and more like a majestic honey badger—a honey badger living its best life. Being screen-free can encourage you to engage with life and activities that you enjoy, like taking a dance class, kicking ass in BJJ, or chasing butterflies in the park like an eight-year-old who still believes in magic.

Limiting exposure to social media can help you avoid the dreaded "comparison-itis" and reduce feelings of anxiety and FOMO (fear of missing out). Instead, it can give you more time to connect with people face-to-face, like your grandma, childhood best friend, or new crush. When you disconnect, you will experience a sense of calm and have space for self-reflection, leading to improved emotional regulation and stress management. It's like taking a mental bubble bath—it might not solve all your problems, but it sure feels nice. Taking a break from digital devices and social media can be a great act of self-care. So, if you're feeling overwhelmed, anxious, or just plain burnt out, it might be time to take a step back and give yourself a digital detox. Give your brain the spa day it deserves and unplug. Your mind and body will thank you, and who knows, you might even discover that your best life exists outside of your social media stories.

Start by setting some boundaries for yourself. Maybe it's no phones at the dinner table, no screens in the bedroom, or taking a day off social media each week. Find what works for you and stick to it. Then fill your time with activities that make you feel good.

Take a yoga class, go for a walk in nature, or spend time with loved ones.

Remember, self-care is not selfish; it's necessary for your well-being. Please be kind to yourself. We all have days where we spend a little too much time scrolling through Instagram or binge-watching Netflix. Don't beat yourself up about it; just recognize it, identify what you learned from the experience, commit to something different, and move on.

TAKE YOUR SUPPLEMENTS

There are some basic supplements I recommend everyone take. Maybe not every day forever, but regularly enough to protect you from the daily stress, inflammation, and toxic assaults on your body.

- **Methylated B Complex** - B vitamins are my number one and most favorite supplements because they feed your mitochondria and help with detoxification, methylation, hormone, and neurotransmitter production.

- **Multiple Minerals** - Minerals are necessary cofactors for basically every process in your body, and our soils aren't as replete with minerals as they once were due to corporate farming practices. You can't get optimal levels from food. Anyone who tells you differently isn't paying attention.

- **Magnesium glycinate** - For sleep, detox, hormones, and neurotransmitter production. This is my preferred form of magnesium because it is highly absorbable and also provides glycine, which helps with detoxification and relaxation. Magnesium threonate is great for people experiencing anxiety and depression, so you can experiment with both.

- **Probiotic** - I like to rotate probiotics because, no matter what Viome says, no one has any idea what the optimal microbiome is except your body when you are doing the things that you need to do to optimize your health. That is why exercise, mindfulness, and fiber are great additions to a wellness program; they support your body in its own personal, ideal microbiome balance.

- **Liver Support** - My favorite liver herbs are milk thistle, dandelion, burdock, and turmeric. The active constituents that support the liver aren't water-soluble, so liver-supportive teas don't help with detox. Get a good supplement and take it daily to combat your daily toxicants.

- **Vitamin C** - When you stress an animal in a laboratory setting, their production of vitamin C skyrockets to insulate them from that stress. You can't make vitamin C, so take it.

- **Essential Fatty Acids** - from either fish or algae because only roughly 10 percent of people can adequately convert plant-based fatty acids (ALA) like those found in avocados, olives, and nuts to the forms we need, EPA and DHA. I haven't seen a single person in my clinical practice who didn't have an impairment here in their genome. This is yet another reason vegans are so often ill. If you choose algae-based forms, check the dosages because you want about 1200mg of omega-3s a day. That means roughly twice as many pills if it's from algae. Under no circumstances should you take krill oil; it isn't worth the money and is endangering the balance of the planet.

- **Vitamin D and K** - These fat-soluble vitamins are important for tissue integrity and the immune system.

- **Iodine** - It is needed for metabolism and immune system function.

Soils are depleted, fruits and vegetables are picked before they are ripe so they can withstand shipping from all over the world, and then they are exposed to ethylene gas to artificially ripen them. Even if you are eating local, organic, seasonal produce, you aren't getting enough nutrients from food in large enough amounts to replenish deficiencies. If you want to make large deposits of nutrients into your health bank account, supplementation is critical. You can then maintain optimal levels by homesteading in western Montana, Costa Rica, or the Mongolian steppe—somewhere relatively free of pollution with nutrient-dense soils. You can visit https://projects.propublica.org/toxmap/ and search your zip code to see if you are in an area of elevated cancer risk due to air pollution from local industry. Check https://www.ewg.org/tapwater/ for a list of toxicants in your water and their possible health impacts.

Like my brilliant, sarcastic brother says:

"Sure. Don't take supplements; you are only breathing, eating and drinking toxicants every moment of every day."
~Dr. Garrett Wdowin

These are the basic supplements I recommend taking daily. You can certainly go down the rabbit hole with optimal supplementation protocols built on your genome and micronutrient testing. You can visit my website for more information on other protocols for fatigue, hormone imbalances, detoxification, autoimmunity, cardiovascular and metabolic issues, anxiety, depression, migraines,and digestive issues, or to get a personalized plan to optimize your health and wellness based on functional medical testing. The Wilde Vitality Detoxification Program has a supplement plan that accompanies it to optimize the removal of toxicants and toxins from your body as well.

THE DR. WILDE WHEEL

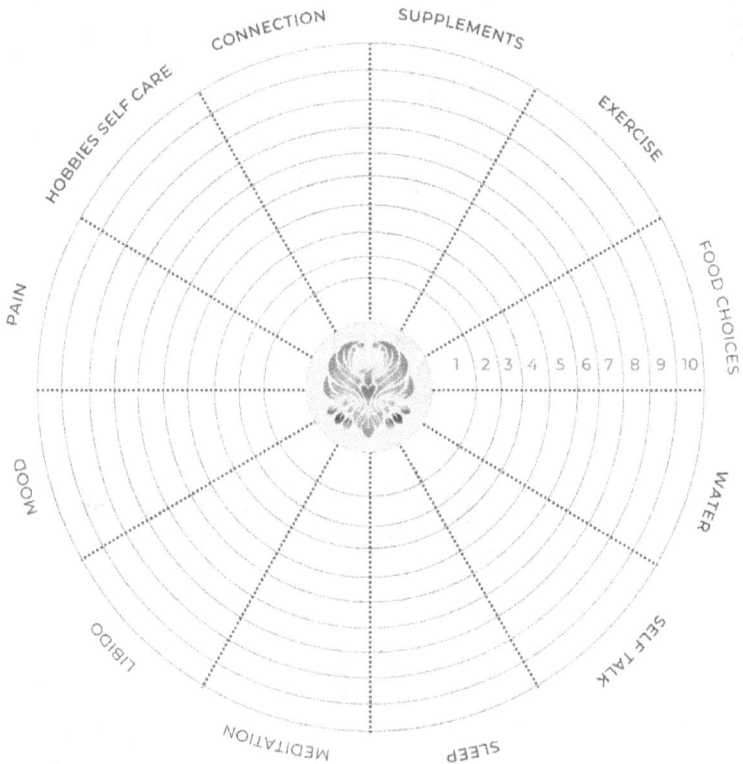

I created this version of a life coaching wheel to specifically support holistic health processes and create awareness of where you can make changes to optimize your health and vitality.

Rate your level of satisfaction in each area: Use a scale of 1–10 to rate how satisfied you currently are in each area listed, or how well you think you are doing what needs to be done to create health. Mark each section of the wheel with a dot or line at the corresponding number.

Connect the dots: Once you have marked your satisfaction levels in each area, connect the dots to create a visual representation of your Wilde Wheel. This will give you a quick overview of which areas of your life need more attention.

Use the information from your Dr. Wilde Wheel to set goals and take action in the areas of your life that need improvement. You may want to use it in conjunction with The Wilde Life Planner, a life or health coach, or a counselor to help you create a plan of action and hold you accountable for making progress.

MINDFULLY CREATE HABITS

The more you participate in a behavior, the more likely it is to become a habit. Think about adding these behaviors to your AM and PM regimens. I created The Wilde Life Planner to support the creation of healthy habits so you too can live your best life by shining awareness on where you can improve and how to choose your health adventure. Be intentional, pay attention, be brave enough to make changes, and create your best life.

CHAPTER 20
DON'T FORGET VITAMIN N

The further we get from nature, the more ill we become. Toxicants stress and damage our bodies. We wake up too early and go to bed too late. Screens provide artificial light and artificial social connections. Virtual reality goggles cause brain damage in children under 12 because they impact how the brain gets wired for depth perception. It is in the warning; if your kids are using them, it might serve you to read the warnings. Not all toxicants are unnatural; mercury and lead, for example, are naturally occurring. They are, however, toxic to life, and their use in manufacturing products has spread them far and wide into the environment. Plastics do not occur in nature, and they don't biodegrade back into it.

Packaged food is often not even recognizable as food. Artificial preservatives keep food longer, so it is resistant to the natural processes of degradation and rot. Think about the Twinkie mythos. Artificial flavors are designed to mimic the taste of natural flavors at a lower production cost. Artificial colors and sweeteners try to take shortcuts around calories and camouflage poor quality by enhancing appearance. The trick is on you; artificial sweeteners still have an insulin response, leading to insulin resistance and prediabetes, and the colors have negative effects on behavior because they are neurotoxic.

That is why I recommend eating the way that I do: natural, unprocessed, organic foods are always better for the body. There is nothing made in a lab by the hubris of humanity that is more beneficial to put in your mouth than something that evolved over millions of years to interact with our genetics and metabolism. Getting closer to nature through natural ingredients makes your body stronger and more vital every time.

In addition to natural ingredients and foods, being in a natural environment supports optimal health. Sleep-wake cycles and paying attention to your circadian rhythm are important parts of being in tune with nature. People who work night shifts and go against their natural sleep rhythms have a life expectancy ten years lower than those who work day shifts. They have a 38% higher risk of dying from cardiovascular disease and a 33% higher risk of dying from colon cancer simply because they go against nature and are awake at night.

Natural foods and rhythms aren't the only health-supporting aspects of nature. In today's fast-paced and technology-driven world, we often find ourselves disconnected from nature, surrounded by the artificial and the fake.

Immersing yourself in a natural environment has been shown to have numerous health benefits for both physical and mental well-being. Whether it's a hike in the woods, a day at the beach, or simply spending time in your local park, being in a natural environment has a positive impact on your overall health.

Exposure to forests and trees has documented health benefits. Research has shown that being among trees and spending time in forests reduces stress. By reducing stress, you are decreasing the impacts of one of the main drivers of chronic disease and can experience accelerated recovery from surgery or illness, increased energy levels, improved sleep, immune system boosts, and lowered blood pressure. Forest exposure improves brain function, resulting in an improved mood and increased ability to focus, even in children with ADHD.

Being in nature has been shown to improve cognitive function, including memory, attention, and creativity. Studies have found that exposure to natural environments can increase blood flow to the brain, which can help improve cognitive function.

Even looking at pictures of nature had similar stress-busting and brain-supporting effects. But why not optimize the experience? The Japanese coined the term "forest bathing," or shinrin-yoku, in the 1980s, and it improves overall well-being. Forest bathing involves spending time in a forest or other natural environment, immersing oneself in the surroundings, and engaging with nature through all the senses.

This practice has been shown to have significant benefits for both physical and mental health. One of the reasons that forest bathing is so effective is that it provides a break from the constant stimulation of modern life. Spending time in nature can help us disconnect from our social media accounts, negative, fear-mongering media outlets, phones, computers, and other devices and allow us to focus on the present moment. This can help reduce feelings of overwhelm and improve our ability to focus.

Another reason that forest bathing is so effective is that it engages all of the senses. Unlike other forms of therapy or exercise, forest bathing involves not just physical activity but also engagement with the natural environment through sight, sound, touch, taste, and smell. This multi-sensory experience can be deeply relaxing and rejuvenating. When was the last time you fully immersed yourself in an experience? When did you engage with all your senses and concentrate on the present moment? You may not have even been fully engaged the last time you had sex!

Your mind is elsewhere– chattering away about the meaningless: *"Hmmmmmm, what am I going to wear tomorrow?"*

There are many ways to incorporate nature into your life. You can go for a walk in a local park or nature reserve, take a hike in a nearby forest, or simply spend some time sitting outside and enjoying being alive—breathing the air, feeling the sun on your skin, and listening to the birds sing. It's important to be mindful and present during your time in nature and to engage all of your senses.

Just being outside in a natural environment has been shown to improve moods and increase feelings of happiness. Exposure to sunlight and fresh air can help boost serotonin levels, which is the hormone responsible for regulating mood. In addition, the greenery and natural beauty of the environment can have a positive impact on our emotional state.

Spending time in nature can also have physical health benefits. Walking or hiking in nature is a great form of exercise—way better than an artificial, germ-ridden gym—and can help improve cardiovascular health, increase endurance, and build muscle. Additionally, exposure to sunlight can help boost vitamin D levels, which are important for maintaining healthy bones and a strong immune system.

Nature is a great anti-inflammatory and can help reduce inflammation in the body. Remember, chronic inflammation has been linked to many horrific health conditions, including heart disease, diabetes, and cancer. Being in a natural environment can help reduce inflammation by decreasing the production of inflammatory markers in the body.

As a functional medicine and naturopathic physician, I have a deep appreciation for the interconnectedness of humanity and nature. I believe that nature is not just a source of beauty and wonder but also a powerful ally in promoting health and well-being.

When we spend time outside, we are not just enjoying the fresh air and beautiful scenery. We are also engaging in a form of therapy that has been shown to have numerous health benefits.

Health is not just the absence of disease but a state of optimal wellness that encompasses every aspect of our lives. This includes our relationship with nature. When we connect with the natural world, we are tapping into a source of healing and renewal that has been part of the human experience for millennia. Your body is a marvel of existence and will heal itself if you give it what it needs and stop doing what is damaging it.

NATUROPATHIC MEDICINE

Naturopathic physicians put "nature" into medicine. We are the experts in preventative, functional, alternative, and holistic medicine because we are trained as primary care doctors with the same coursework and study of anatomy, physiology, pathology, biochemistry, microbiology, diagnostics, and pharmacology as MDs and DOs.

Then, we also study botanical medicine, acupuncture, nutrition, orthomolecular supplementation, physical medicine, exercise therapy, counseling, environmental medicine, homeopathy, mind-body medicine, and how those therapeutics can apply to everything that can go wrong with a human being's body and all the medical specialties from pain management to oncology. It's a lot of education.

We are also guided by the following philosophical tenets that support health, wellness, and vitality:

PRIMUM, NON NOCERE: FIRST, DO NO HARM

One of the more famous phrases of the Hippocratic oath is "do no harm." I don't believe sane healthcare providers want to hurt their patients. I do believe they are often unable to implement effective therapies in a preventative manner to reverse disease due to politics and corporate agendas. Just like omissions can be seen as lying, not giving alternatives to toxic therapies and dangerous surgeries due to outside influences could be interpreted as "harming."

Sometimes I daydream about going to law school so I can write cease and desist letters to providers who tell patients there's "no research" on a supplement or alternative therapy when, in fact, they just haven't looked at the research. My mentor wrote a book with thousands of peer-reviewed studies showing the efficacy of alternative therapies for cancer. Another example is the fact that CoQ10 production in your body is seriously inhibited by HMG-CoA reductase inhibitors, or statin drugs.

That is physiology and doesn't need a research study. If you aren't taking a CoQ10 supplement with a statin, you are depriving your body of a powerful antioxidant and important fuel for your mitochondria. Even the Mayo Clinic recognizes the efficacy of CoQ10 supplementation for congestive heart failure and high cholesterol in diabetes. Surprisingly, many providers don't recommend this supplement to the patients they prescribe statins to, nor do they recognize its value. In my opinion, that is harmful, and *"Ignorantia physiologia non excusat."* Ignorance of physiology is no excuse.

PREVENIRE: PREVENTION

Prevention is an essential component of modern medicine, offering a range of benefits beyond just financial savings on future heroic medical interventions like quadruple bypass and organ replacement. By adopting healthy behaviors and creating supportive environments, we can effectively mitigate the risk factors associated with chronic diseases and promote overall wellness.

One of the key advantages of prevention is its efficacy in improving health outcomes. By adopting healthy habits such as regular exercise, a balanced diet, regenerative sleep, a positive mindset, and detoxification, we can significantly reduce the incidence of chronic conditions such as cardiovascular disease, stroke, and cancer. Furthermore, creating environments that promote healthy lifestyles can help reinforce these behaviors, contributing to sustained health improvements and a better chance that you will be able to live your best life.

TOLLE CAUSAM: TREAT THE CAUSE

A "green allopath" could give a natural substance like melatonin instead of a prescription sleeping pill and still not treat the cause of the disease. Holistic providers of any value will investigate your labs, health history, and clinical picture to determine what is causing your illness or unwanted symptoms and then treat that cause. For example, if you are on screens late at night, it is impacting your sleep and resulting in insomnia. Or if you are eating too many carbs, that could be one layer of the cause of your prediabetes. Functional medicine providers will dig deeper and see why you are experiencing health declines. There is a reason beyond *"You are just getting older,"* and we are trained to find it.

TOLLE TOTUM: TREAT THE WHOLE PERSON

As I discussed in the first section of this book, a human is so much more than one organ system or even just the body. Stress, for example, is a mental, emotional, and physical reaction to the environment, and just addressing the effect of stress on the body isn't as effective as supporting the mental and emotional as well as decreasing the environmental exposure to that stress. The best medical providers will not only find and treat the cause of the disease; they will also treat all aspects of you in your healing process. That is the definition of "holistic medicine."

DOCERE: DOCTOR AS TEACHER

Today, a new client asked me what working with me would be like. I replied that I aimed to educate and empower him about what was going on in his body, to work with him to shine the light on what his body needed to heal, and to share my experience and expertise with him so that he could make the best choices for his own body on his personal health adventure.

How many times have you heard that knowledge is power? It may be a well-worn adage, but it is nonetheless true. A restriction on knowledge is disempowering. When information is hidden from you or made too complicated for you to understand, how are you able to make informed decisions about your most precious possession, the health of your body? Do you understand why the last lab tests your doctor ordered were done, and do you know what the levels meant? Were they explained to you? If you have been prescribed medications, do you know what they do in your body and their possible side effects? Have you been educated about the potential causes of your symptoms or disease?

If you were better informed about what was affecting your health, would you make different choices? If you knew that something you were eating was making you sick, would you stop eating it? If you knew that using a certain household cleaner made your autoimmunity worse, would you find an alternative? If you knew that your body was low in vitamin D, would you take it?

VIX MEDICATRIX NATURAE: THE HEALING POWER OF NATURE

Often, this phrase is interpreted as referring to using herbs and supplements rather than pharmaceuticals. There is something called "green allopathy," a phenomenon when people who want to move more toward alternative medicine substitute a "natural" substance for a drug rather than finding and treating the cause of the disease.

For example, red rice yeast has a similar biochemical action in the body as a statin drug; both substances inhibit the production of cholesterol in the liver. One can be patented and is therefore a prescription, and one cannot because, at this time, natural substances still cannot be patented, and so is an over-the-counter supplement.

I interpret the "healing power of nature" as what is inherently happening in your body and being when you align your consumption and habits with those more in line with natural processes, in addition to using natural elements to support health and healing. The power that moves your body toward health is called the "Vis." It is the power that animates us and is part of the mystery of what "life" is. It is the force that moves the body toward wellness. How do we heal a cut without thinking about it? We just have to stop cutting ourselves and give the body what it needs to repair itself. That process is not different from how true physicians can support you in treating diabetes or allergies.

Nature itself is a complex entity made up of many organisms and ecosystems. I believe that our connection to nature is fundamental to our health and well-being. By spending time outside, we can tap into a powerful source of healing and renewal that has sustained humanity for centuries. And by caring for the environment, we can ensure that this healing power is available for generations to come.

So let us embrace the beauty and wonder of nature and work together to promote health, wellness, and sustainability for all. Our connection to nature is not just about the benefits we receive. It is also our responsibility to care for the natural world. As a functional medicine doctor and naturopathic physician, I understand that our health is intimately linked to the health of the planet. We cannot separate ourselves from the environment in which we live. Our choices and actions have a profound impact on the world around us.

So, I encourage you to spend time outside, connect

with nature, and teach your children to value the natural world. I also encourage you to be mindful of your impact on the environment, choose your products wisely, reduce waste and conserve resources, support sustainable practices, and protect wildlife. Don't throw soup on art masterpieces; all that does is feed disrespect and negativity. If you are not outraged, however, you aren't paying attention. You can go back to TikTok cat videos and live a life of quiet desperation, or you can take action to defend yourself, your family, and your home.

The East Palestine, Ohio, train derailment happened while I was putting the finishing touches on this book. Politicians often run on platforms supposedly supporting the environment, and where are they now? Who is advocating for the people impacted by that spill? We are all affected by toxicity, so who is responsible for your health issues that are driven by toxicity? Is DuPont going to pay for your medical bills? For your children's cancer or infertility treatments?

Toxicity isn't contained within a state or country; our water tables and air currents are all connected. Who is going to speak for us—for you, your children, and your grandchildren, who aren't expected to live as long as you? Do you believe that the government and corporations have your best interests in mind?

I don't. Every aspect of your health is under attack. Your food, water, and air are all poisoned. Your personal care and household products are poisoned. Your government is no longer a republic for the people and by the people; a study from Princeton showed it is a corporate oligarchy that serves the interests of the companies that have taken over your government departments. Big Ag owns the USDA. Big

Pharma owns the FDA and the CDC. Big Oil and Big Chem own the EPA. These are the departments that were designed to protect you, and they are now serving corporate interests. Your economy is stressed, inflation is rampant, and we are under threat of a world war. Your culture is sick, and your social networks are being eroded and replaced with fantasy. Your education and social services have been systematically defunded to create a populace that lacks agency and support and turns to pharmaceutical options to manage their uncomfortable emotions that threaten to drown them.

Creating your best life is completely up to you. Choose your health and life's adventures wisely. I believe we can work together to care for the planet and promote health for ourselves and future generations by voting with our dollars and living with integrity and respect for this beautiful planet.

Hold polluters accountable by not buying their goods and connecting with others in meaningful ways because no matter what color or pronouns, religion, or political affiliation we are, we all have red blood, are subject to the laws of physics and physiology, and are being poisoned by chemical toxicants. Social media may be a soul-sucking, malignant pimple on the buttocks of the 21st-century human experience, but it is also a powerful tool when used with intention. Join me on social media and help me support transformative conversations that will serve us all.

Knowledge is power, and there is great strength in banding together, communicating with open minds and hearts, educating one another, finding alternatives to toxic products, sharing them, and speaking out. Take action. Your health and life depend on it.

www.ingramcontent.com/pod-product-compliance
Lightning Source LLC
Chambersburg PA
CBHW052127270326
41930CB00012B/2783